Leading Antenatal Classes

A practical guide

To all parents – past, present and future

Leading Antenatal Classes

A practical guide

Judy Priest and Judith Schott

Illustrations by Helen Chown BA(Hons) Fine Art

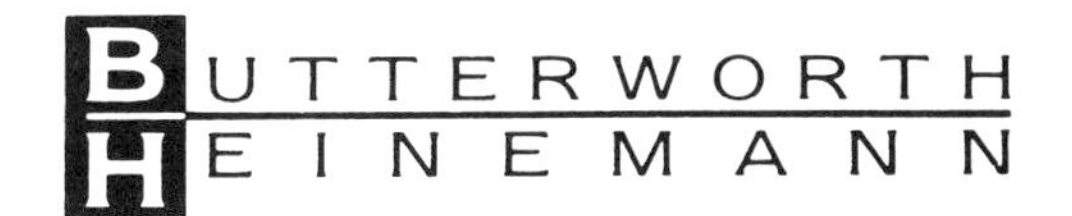

Butterworth-Heinemann
Linacre House, Jordan Hill, Oxford OX2 8DP
A division of Reed Educational and Professional Publishing Ltd

A member of the Reed Elsevier plc group

OXFORD BOSTON JOHANNESBURG
MELBOURNE NEW DELHI SINGAPORE

First published 1991
Reprinted 1991, 1993, 1994, 1996, 1997

British Library Cataloguing in Publication Data
Priest, Judy
Leading antenatal classes.
I. Title II. Schott, Judith
618.20028

ISBN 0 7506 0050 0

Library of Congress Cataloging in Publication Data
Priest, Judy.
Leading antenatal classes: a practical guide/Judy Priest and Judith Schott.
p. cm.
Includes bibliographical references and index.
ISBN 0 7506 0050 0
1. Childbirth—Study and teaching. I. Schott, Judith.
II. Title.
[DNLM: 1. Patient Education—methods. 2. Prenatal Care. WQ 175 P9491]
RG973.P75 1991
618.2'4'0715—dc20
DNLM/DLC 91-29288
for Library of Congress CIP

Composition by Genesis Typesetting, Laser Quay, Rochester, Kent
Printed in Great Britain by St Edmundsbury Press Limited, Bury St Edmunds, Suffolk

Contents

Foreword vii

Acknowledgements viii

Introduction 1

Part I The potential of antenatal education 5

1 The changes that pregnancy brings 7
2 What do parents want from classes? 10
3 How people learn 12
4 Exploring why teachers run classes 17
Further reading 23

Part II The basics of an antenatal course 25

5 Planning a course 27
6 Getting started 39
7 Giving information 53
8 Communicating effectively 63
9 Leading discussion 71
10 Encouraging active learning 82
11 Teaching physical skills 95
12 Relaxation 100
13 Breathing, massage, positions and exercise 114
14 Visual aids 133
15 Team-teaching 147
Further reading 152

Part III Fine-tuning your antenatal course 155

16 Preparing for parenthood 157
17 Working with fathers 161
18 Groups with shared needs 170
19 Handling difficult topics 188
20 Being an agent for change 198
Further reading 203

Part IV Thinking about you and your teaching 207

21 You and your teaching: self-assessment and skills assessment 209
22 Trying out new approaches 219
23 Setting up a working partnership 221
24 Ongoing training 227

Appendix I Addresses of organizations 231

Appendix II Visual aids addresses 237

Index 239

Foreword

I am pleased to be associated with this visionary work of Judy and Judith for teachers of antenatal classes.

- It offers new, and experienced teachers, opportunities to explore and evaluate approaches to various aspects of antenatal preparation for expectant parents.
- It offers a reminder of the fundamental effects pregnancy has on the social and working lives and relationships of expectant parents, their families and friends.
- It offers pragmatic counsel drawn from years of practical acquaintance with this important facet of preparation for parenthood.
- It offers a framework for teachers to recognize and meet their own needs with an emphasis on support, reflection and evaluation.

Within the maternity services a high degree of physical safety for women and babies is achievable. The challenge now is to gain further improvements in outcomes, in areas of morbidity and the satisfaction and involvement of women in care. More attention to the provision of social, psychological and educative support for women and their partners is an essential component of achieving further improvements.

In sharing their experiences the authors of this book show how it is possible to provide sensitive antenatal preparation, involving prospective parents throughout, whilst revealing their deep commitment and humour.

This must be an urgent first step in meeting the challenge. Read the book – take up the summons!

Maternity Services Manager/ Director of Midwifery Services University College Hospital London

Anne C. E. Rider RN, RM, MTD

Acknowledgements

This book reflects what we have learned about antenatal teaching and about ourselves as teachers. Many people have contributed to our development and understanding and we are deeply appreciative of them all.

First and foremost, our thanks go to Nancy James and Veronica Taylor, our colleagues in PROSPECT. Through setting up this partnership and working together designing and running workshops for health professionals, we constantly learn from each other. We laugh a lot, cry occasionally and have fun together. Over the years, our combined ideas and pooled experiences have produced what is recorded here. On every page, this book reflects the PROSPECT approach.

We would also like to thank others who have commented on the text and listened while we sorted out our thoughts and worked through the sticky patches. These include Alix Henley whose shrewd comments and encouragement have been invaluable, Pip Wilcox and Lesley Marks who are always ready to listen, Jill Gingell and Margaret Beavis for their support and interest and Anne Rider who commented on the text as well as writing the Foreword. Thanks are also due to Nancy Kline for helping to crystallize our ideas on working partnerships. The final responsibility for what is here, however, rests with us.

Our thanks, too, to our families for being patient and understanding while we sat in front of word processors and had long phone calls with each other. Benjamin deserves a special mention for the many times he came to the rescue when the machines wouldn't do what we wanted.

Above all, we would like to express our deep appreciation for all the expectant parents who have come to our classes, the colleagues who have shared their ideas, and all the health professionals and lay teachers who have attended our workshops and tutorials.

Introduction

Each person attending antenatal classes is unique. Each brings her or his own blend of experience, needs and expectations and will take away different things. In the same way, we anticipate that each person who reads this book, whatever their level of experience or knowledge, will respond differently to it and will choose or refuse, change or use the suggestions we offer.

We chose the title *Leading Antenatal Classes* carefully to reflect our philosophy and practice. We believe that participants are best served by a sensitive leader who develops and maintains a creative learning environment. A teacher in the strict dictionary definition of the word is 'one who instructs' and no one denies the need for giving information. But so much more than instruction goes on when a class works together, talks together and gets to know each other. To achieve all they can in a class, expectant parents need to operate as a group, not a passive audience awaiting instruction.

So what should the person running the class be called? No single word quite sums up the role, so for the sake of clarity we decided to stick with 'teacher' rather than 'leader' or 'facilitator'. A true teacher is someone who educates in the original sense of the word, that is 'one who draws out' or 'leads forth' rather than puts in. With apologies to men who teach classes we refer to the teacher as 'she' rather than 'he'.

The second half of our title – A Practical Guide – reflects the second characteristic of the book. It is about the *process* of antenatal teaching – how to start a group, how to get people talking, how to share information, how to teach relaxation. We also include ways of reaching decisions about *content* – what to include in the course. However, there are as many different ways of putting a course together as there are teachers, and different groups will have different needs. Your own experience and your knowledge of the needs of the people you teach are your best guides in helping you decide which facts to cover, which topics to include and which particular skills parents will find useful.

You will notice as you read that, like an effective antenatal class, this book includes overlap and repetition. Issues don't fit into separate boxes labelled 'groupwork' or 'discussion' or 'visual aids'. For example, when you are starting a group, you need to keep in mind various thoughts about how groups work, how the physical surroundings affect the group, and what support you yourself need to lead the group well. These factors are just as important when you are teaching pelvic floor exercises or touring the hospital delivery room. Topics, too, can flow into one another in an infinite variety of new and exciting combinations. So while we have divided up the material into separate subjects, we often invite you to refer to other chapters as you read. One advantage of this is that you end up looking at a topic from several different perspectives.

You may also notice that we frequently mention men. This may seem unnecessary since women make up the majority of class participants and many are not supported by a partner either during pregnancy or in antenatal classes. It may also seem presumptuous. As women, we know how we feel when men speak on our behalf. However, men become parents too. Most of what we know about fathers and partners we learned from men who were willing to talk openly about their experiences and feelings. If you are a woman and find it hard to put yourself into the shoes of men, some of the approaches we suggest could help you gain new insights into their needs in relation to childbearing and parenthood.

There is always more that one could put into an antenatal course than there is room for. In the same way we have had to make hard decisions about how much to include and how much to leave out. Many of the topics we address merit a whole book to themselves. You will find books that do concentrate on particular issues included in the Further Reading lists placed at the end of each of the four parts of the book.

The issues we do include do not add up to a hard-and-fast recipe for running classes. Each class is made up of individuals and both you and they are dealing with ever-changing situations and a constant flow of new information. You cannot even be sure that what worked last time will work the next. However, you can become more skilled and able to work confidently with whatever happens.

Whatever your interest or level of experience, we suggest you start by reading Part I, in which we discuss the more philosophical aspects of antenatal education. Then dip into the practical chapters in Parts II and III, selecting those that are of particular relevance to you and the people you are teaching. Before you put any new approaches into practice, we suggest you read Part IV, which looks at the business of antenatal teaching from the teacher's perspective and focuses on the importance of looking after yourself.

Everything we describe in this book reflects the experience and observations we have gathered over many years of teaching antenatal classes and of working with health professionals and lay people involved in antenatal education. We do not include statistics or research studies to support what we offer, although sources are included in the lists of suggested reading. Here is what we have tried and tested and found to work in practice.

Part I

The potential of antenatal education

1

The changes that pregnancy brings

Any pregnancy, but most especially the first one, is a life crisis. It is a time of heightened awareness and great change. Parents begin to see themselves, each other and the world differently. During the nine months it takes for a baby to grow, parents develop and grow too, so that one year later almost nothing in the parents' lives remains as it was before the baby was conceived.

Physical changes are perhaps most evident and a woman has little choice but to take notice of them. This may be a new experience, because although most women work hard to try to ensure that their appearance conforms with current fashion and social images, many pay little real heed to their bodies. Other changes are just as intrusive and unavoidable as the growing baby forces parents to review every aspect of their lifestyles. Some are relatively trivial but may still be hard to cope with. What to wear as the woman's shape changes? Is it safe for her to continue riding her bike? What about holidays? Wine? Discotheques? Others are more central as they concern work, money or housing issues: 'Can we afford to live here?' 'Is there room for a baby?' 'Who gives up work or do we need two incomes?' 'What about the rising damp?' 'Will the council give us a flat now?'

Even the structure of a woman's day changes. Tiredness may force her to bed early. Broken nights and vivid dreams may find her awake at unusual times. Giving up work, even temporarily, is a major step for many women. It may be a relief, but it may also create anxieties about loss of status, loss of income or worries about arranging suitable child care if the woman plans to return to work. Enforced leisure leaves many women at a loss and unsure of how to structure their days.

Not just practical issues, but ideas and feelings also change. Pregnancy often seems to take the 'emotional lid' off, allowing both women and men to become more sensitive, aware and in touch with their deeper feelings. Women tend to laugh and cry more easily, while many men feel anxious and unsettled.

Some women cope with all the changes of pregnancy on their own, but most share the experience with a partner. The demands that pregnancy makes on a father are often unrecognized and unacknowledged because nothing visible is happening to him. However, his world is changing too, as he adapts to the physical and emotional changes in his partner and to the financial, practical and emotional responsibilities that fatherhood brings.

Society casts a father in the dual roles of supporter and breadwinner, but offers little understanding of the changes these new roles bring. These changes affect each individual in different ways. For some men, the impending arrival of a baby threatens the exclusive relationship they have with their partner. They are no longer the sole focus of her attention and care. Other men, who long for fatherhood and for direct contact with their child, can find the pregnancy long and frustrating. And many men worry about the safety of their partner and child.

When expectant parents change, those around them must change too. Other family members will also be making adjustments. A couple's parents may welcome or hate the idea of becoming grandparents. Some are supportive and encouraging. Others may be critical, offering inappropriate advice or unwanted opinions. Some have difficulty in acknowledging that their child is now an adult who has a demonstrably active sex life and will make his or her own decisions about the coming baby. Other family members will also be affected. They may welcome or resent the couple's changing status and lifestyle. Whatever the attitudes, parents need to work out new ways of relating to familiar people.

Expectant parents often reassess their friendships. Friends who have no children and lead a busy social life may not understand the exhaustion some pregnant women feel, or may be bored by talk of birth and babies. Those who have babies or small children can become sources of support and act as models for prospective parents who are beginning to think about how they will handle the countless problems they will face. Less helpfully, experienced parents can offer conflicting or intrusive advice. Friends are often work colleagues and whether a woman returns to work or not, the changes brought about by the pregnancy and arrival of the baby will inevitably alter these relationships.

It's little wonder that after a few months of experiencing a combination of novelty, unpredictability and discomfort, expectant parents begin to wonder what has hit them. Where is the familiar world and their familiar part in it? Where, even, is the body they used to know? Nine months can seem endless, but it is really quite a short time in which to develop ways of coping with so much that is new.

Prospective parents adjust and manage in all kinds of ways. Some carry on as if nothing much is happening and try to maintain life as it was before. Others seem to focus entirely on the coming baby. They may read anything they can lay their hands on, talk to experienced people, or live for their check-ups. One common strategy for coping with the changes and challenges of pregnancy is to attend antenatal classes. These offer the couple another avenue towards understanding more about what is currently happening and prepare them for what is to come.

Most people who make the effort to come along to classes have high hopes about what they might gain from them. Happily, the same combination of factors that drives expectant parents to seek out classes – uncertainty, changing perceptions of themselves and their world, and hunger for information – also fosters a climate for learning that is unique in most adults' lives. During pregnancy, parents are adapting physically and emotionally to take on what is probably the greatest responsibility of their lives. Because of rapid change and an uncertain future, they are open to feelings and ideas. Many are searching for information and all of them need to feel cherished and cared for.

2

What do parents want from classes?

If you ask expectant parents in the first week of an antenatal course why they have come, they give many answers: 'To find out more', 'To meet people', 'Because I worry about everything', 'To learn how to care for a new baby', 'To meet the staff'. Their responses are likely to be varied and fairly straightforward.

But these initial responses may not be the whole story. As people become more confident, they may offer additional, more complicated explanations. Perhaps they came because their friends did or because it felt like the right thing to do. Some people fear that *not* coming would be in some way neglecting their baby or maybe even tempting fate. Many hope for a magic formula to make labour safe and painless or that classes will help the father to be supportive during labour.

Often, participants themselves will be unaware of all their motives. Although many women know that they have come to meet other pregnant women who share their experiences and preoccupations, they may be less aware that they are also looking for behaviour patterns they can copy or useful information they can tap. Antenatal classes may be the only place they can find these things, since in everyday life, contact with pregnant women, expectant fathers or young babies is fairly unusual until one's own first baby is born.

Another underlying reason for coming to classes is to find family substitutes, especially if the parents' own extended family lives far away or if relationships are difficult. Even when family bonds are strong, rapid changes in midwifery and obstetric practice limit the amount of information and shared experiences relatives can offer. In areas where continuity of care has yet to be introduced, once classes start, the antenatal teacher may be the only person who is constant, available and willing to talk and listen. She may take on the role of an experienced woman, able to act as ally, supportive friend and information source.

It is not only interesting to find out why people come, it is also important. If you understand what people want, you can help them to separate achievable from unattainable goals and think about what they can realistically expect. You can also adapt your course in response to their needs and expectations. Chapter 6 suggests a variety of ways to find out why people have come.

Past experiences of learning

Parents' expectations of antenatal classes are shaped by many things. One important factor is their own past experiences of learning. These will be as varied as the people who come. Those who have been successful at the kind of learning which consisted of amassing and remembering facts often see birth and parenthood as another test to pass or fail. They may want clear-cut information and a defined set of actions to follow which will produce the desired effect. There will usually be others in the group who found schooling competitive and learning difficult. They may have an aversion to being taught or being put into any situation where there is a 'right' or a 'wrong' answer. Often, such people are anxious that their worst memories of school might be repeated in the class. Still other people will be deferential and anxious to please, while a few will be suspicious or even antagonistic.

Each expectant parent comes with her or his own personal history and individual hopes and fears. The challenge for you, the teacher, is to encourage all these people – the keen, the worried and the reluctant – to acquire new skills and knowledge. You are more likely to do this well if you have an understanding of how people learn. The next chapter suggests ways to use what is known about how people learn to the best advantage in your classes.

3

How people learn

Effective learning enables people to change. It equips us to do things and to respond to situations and challenges in new ways.

We are born with an enormous enthusiasm and capacity to learn. You have only to watch babies and very young children to see that human beings are inherently alert and deeply interested in and inquisitive about themselves, other people and the world around them. This capacity and enthusiasm for learning can be enhanced by positive learning experiences or dampened by negative ones.

- Think about the best teacher or teachers you ever had. Don't restrict yourself to teachers you had at school or during your professional training. Every day we come into contact with a whole variety of people in very different circumstances – some of these may have been the key people from whom you learnt most.
- Now jot down a list of all the qualities, the things they did and said, that made them such a good teacher for you.
- Then think about the worst teachers you ever had and list the things they said and did that made learning difficult.
- Now focus on your learning experiences as an adult. Write down one or two new skills you have acquired in the past couple of years.

What was your motivation for learning these?
What kept you going?
What resources did you use?
What approaches and methods helped you to learn?
Do you absorb information and acquire skills by listening, watching, reading, discussing or experimenting?

Before reading on, take a few minutes to review your own experiences of learning, as suggested in the box opposite. Invite some of your friends and colleagues to do this exercise. Your combined lists will help you identify the different ways that individuals learn and some of the behaviours and attitudes that assist learning. You will also highlight those that are not helpful.

Creating a climate for learning

A great deal is now known about the factors that contribute to a creative learning environment. One of the most readable books we have found is by Jennifer Rogers called *Adults Learning* (see Further Reading at the end of Part I). Using books like this, together with our own beliefs and experience, we have worked out a list of factors that seem most important for us. You may want to add your own or compare what is here with your own list of qualities and factors that have enabled you to learn and which the questions in the box may have generated. You will find a variety of suggestions on how to put these ideals into practice in this book.

The teacher–learner relationship

We now realize that people learn best if the teacher creates opportunities in which people can identify their own needs, play a part in deciding what they will learn and learn in their own ways. This is very different from a teacher transferring a predetermined body of knowledge or skills into passive recipients. Active involvement means the class stops being an audience and starts working as a group of people who interact with the teacher and with each other.

In order for this more mutual relationship to develop, the teacher needs to be caring and involved. This entails going beyond joining in activities or listening to what others say, to being willing to give of herself within the class. By letting participants glimpse your own feelings and thoughts from time to time, you allow them see you as a person rather than someone doing a job.

Clearly it is not appropriate to tell them your life history or details of your own experiences or opinions. You need to find a balance between letting them see you as you are and maintaining boundaries so that you do not dominate or get taken over by the class.

A welcoming environment

In order to learn, people need to feel at ease. They need comfort and privacy in order to relax and focus on the job in hand. This means choosing a room with care or adapting the room you have (see Chapter 6).

Respect and acceptance

Learning means changing and this can feel risky. People's experiences of learning will include memories that are painful or humiliating, leaving many preoccupied with concerns about 'getting it wrong' or 'making a fool of myself'. People will be more able to listen, to think and to try new things if there is an atmosphere of mutual respect and acceptance for every single person in the class whatever his or her knowledge, views, background or lifestyle.

In order to achieve and maintain this atmosphere of respect, you will need to examine your own feelings and attitudes from time to time so that you can treat everyone with acceptance even if you disagree with what they say or do. Part IV has suggestions on how to do this.

Understanding the purpose of learning

People are motivated to learn if they can see some personal relevance or advantage in making the effort. Without this understanding, people may *appear* to comply but their energy and attention will be partly absorbed by wondering, 'What is the point of this?' If you identify and include the things that people say they want from the course, and then take time to establish why they will find it useful to have certain other information and skills, you stimulate people's willingness to learn.

The importance of variety

Research has shown that the average person's attention span is around 20 minutes. After this, people's ability to concentrate and absorb new information declines rapidly. Pregnancy amnesia probably reduces this 20-minute attention span considerably, so it makes sense to vary the pace and change the type of activity frequently throughout each class to get the most from what little time you have.

Variety is also important because each person learns differently. Some learn best by hearing, others are more visual and all need to experiment with new information and skills before they can assimilate and make them their own. By using a variety of approaches, you offer everyone an opportunity to learn in their own particular way.

Building on existing knowledge

People find it easier to grasp a new idea if it relates in some way to something they already understand. By encouraging them to identify what they already know, you boost their self-esteem and build a sound foundation for new skills and knowledge. You, too, will benefit because understanding what they already know helps you to give information in a way that is appropriate to the people with whom you are working.

Welcoming questions and ideas

In order to clarify their ideas, people often need to question or re-state what they have heard in their own words. So encourage questions and comments and treat each and every one with respect. Page 74 suggests ways to trigger questions.

Evaluating and using new knowledge

People need to experiment with new information in order to be able to use it themselves. They do this through discussion. problem-solving or by trying things out for themselves. By allowing time for these activities, you help to ensure effective learning.

Encouragement and affirmation

Success breeds success. Everyone becomes more confident, relaxed and able to learn if each person's contributions and efforts, no matter how small, are appreciated. When people are rewarded with encouragement they will often risk a bigger step in future. Criticism (which usually consists of what is wrong) has the opposite effect on motivation and morale.

Making learning fun

For many of us, learning has been a fraught and serious business, yet fun and learning are not mutually exclusive. Some of the most effective learning and most creative work take place when people are enjoying each other's company and having fun together.

In conclusion

Your classes are made up of a rich mix of individuals. Each one brings expectations, experiences, hopes and fears. By and large, prospective parents are ready and eager to learn. Just occasionally an experienced teacher will meet someone, years later, who says how much the classes meant to them and how they have never forgotten what they learnt. This a rare and precious treat and a graphic reminder of the potential of antenatal classes.

4

Exploring why teachers run classes

There are many different reasons for running antenatal classes and most teachers will have more than one. For some it may be a welcome or unwelcome part of their job. Others may *choose* to lead antenatal classes and may have all kinds of reasons for doing so. Many teach simply because they love it and enjoy being involved with people at a turning point in their lives. Others see it as an opportunity to influence people. Some want others to have as good or better childbearing experiences than they themselves had.

Understanding your motivation

- If you chose to lead antenatal classes, what led you to make that choice?
- If you did not actively choose, but lead classes as part of your job, how do you feel about being in that situation?
- Think through your experiences of caring for parents during pregnancy, labour and the early days after the birth. Are there any particular memories that stand out? What have you found enjoyable and satisfying? What have you found frustrating or difficult?
- If you are a parent, take time to review your own personal experiences of pregnancy, labour and the early days of parenthood. What went well? What did you enjoy or find satisfying? What was hard or difficult?

Each of us needs to understand our motivation for teaching antenatal classes because, however subtly, it affects and influences everything we do. Why are you involved in antenatal teaching? Consider the questions in the box on the previous page and jot down your responses or discuss them with a supportive friend or colleague (see Chapter 23).

For some, past experiences may generate a need to resolve certain issues. There is nothing wrong with having such needs, but since they can influence how people teach, it is probably better to find ways of dealing with them rather than leaving them unrecognized and unresolved. You will find suggestions for tackling these and similar issues in Chapter 21.

Identifying your aims and approach

In addition to your motivation, you will also have things you want to achieve. Unless you clarify your aims, you cannot tell whether or not you are achieving them. Most teachers have a mixture of aims. Here, we discuss three different approaches which grow out of the aims which antenatal teachers usually cite when asked what they are trying to do in classes.

- To influence what people think and do – teaching for persuasion.
- To help people adapt to the system of care they will be offered – teaching for compliance.
- To enable people to make their own choices – teaching for choice.

As you read, you will probably recognize bits of your own style under each heading, since most of us incorporate aspects of several approaches in our courses.

Teaching for persuasion

Influencing what expectant parents think and do can be a teacher's primary aim. This approach has a long history. When parentcraft classes first began, midwifery textbooks of the day contained pictures of midwives with blackboard and chalk giving lectures on balanced diets, baby equipment and the like. It is easy to feel justified in giving strong messages about what a woman should and should not do when her actions will affect not only herself but also the baby she is carrying and will go on nurturing for the next decade or two.

Over the years, our knowledge of what is and is not helpful to growing babies increases and so, too, does the temptation to treat pregnant women as a captive audience for well-intentioned advice. Helping women to stop smoking, to avoid teratogens or to reduce the stress in their lives does bring real benefits to mother and baby. Posture, diet and dental care come under the 'good for you' label, whereas vaccination and effective car restraints are 'good for the baby'.

But there is a catch. Information that does not acknowledge people's circumstances and difficulties is a burden, not an asset. It alienates. So, too, does an implicit message that equates failure to comply with not caring or not being responsible. The additional stress and guilt felt by whoever receives these messages could even accentuate the behaviour the message is designed to change.

Another difficulty with strong messages about self-care is the often tenuous link between knowing something is harmful or beneficial and acting on that knowledge. Most parents know that smoking is harmful to babies but this has not reduced the percentage who smoke. Do you and your colleagues consistently put into practice everything you know is good for your own health?

So where does this leave the teacher who wants to persuade others to change? A pregnant woman's actions *do* matter, because they can affect her dependent, vulnerable baby. Antenatal educators *do* have a duty to provide parents with the information they need to make good decisions for themselves and their growing baby. But information needs to be given in a way that people can hear and act on.

In order to be effective and avoid sounding 'preachy', whoever gives health information must decide which are the key issues to include in the course and which could be omitted. The next step, then, is weaving these messages into the course and bringing them up where they seem to fit best, probably through discussion rather than delivering a lecture. One useful source for ideas for doing this might be the local health promotion department.

The message is more likely to be heard if it is combined with respect, understanding and, if necessary, practical support. After all, changing our habits is hard. If it was easy to give up smoking, eat rationally or limit the use of drugs or alcohol, most people would have done it already. Throughout this book, we discuss ways to help women and their partners feel welcomed, valued and heard, whatever their current behaviour. This can help them build enough self-respect to improve the way they treat themselves.

Another way antenatal teachers can influence parents is to offer them their own personal beliefs and decisions. Expectant parents are anxious, eager for knowledge and unsure of themselves. This vulnerability means that they can be persuaded to adapt their behaviour to match the convictions of a charismatic teacher.

Birth styles or fashions can also be an underlying theme of antenatal classes. Choices range from high-tech obstetrics, 'natural childbirth', or involving siblings in the birth, to excluding men, giving birth under water, or any other approach that the teacher feels justified in encouraging others to embrace.

Classes aimed at persuasion are not propaganda for their own sake. Whatever the particular belief system, persuasive teachers genuinely believe their way is best. A teacher wants parents to benefit from her experience, which often comes from years of practice or work with hundreds of couples. At one level this makes good sense – after all, there is a reason why a professional or trained lay person is running the classes rather than the milkman!

However, shaping what to teach exclusively by personal belief about what is best, offers parents an inaccurate picture of what they are facing. Most firmly held beliefs can be countered by the opposite viewpoint which someone else will hold just as tenaciously: 'Home birth is the best' or 'It's safer in hospital'; 'Labour without an epidural? What's the point of feeling pain?' or 'Drugs for pain mean a second-rate labour and a second-rate start for your baby.' None of these statements is an absolute truth and only individual parents can judge which option is best given the circumstances in which they find themselves. In classes where strong convictions are offered, the teacher may believe she gives others the benefits she herself has found, but in the final analysis this approach benefits the person in charge rather than the parents themselves.

Teaching for compliance

Sometimes, another kind of persuasion is going on in classes. The goal of classes is not to fit parents to the teacher's convictions or to get them to adopt healthier habits; rather, it is to prepare parents for what they will actually meet in labour or on the postnatal ward. This concept of tailoring the course to fit the status quo often generates hot debate when antenatal teachers meet.

What shapes decisions about what to include and what to gloss over? How would you teach your class if, despite the evidence that routine continuous electronic fetal monitoring gives no advantage to many women and babies and is associated with a higher intervention rate, all women will be attached to an electronic fetal monitor? Is there any point in encouraging people to practise a variety of positions so that they can be upright and mobile throughout labour, if you know that in practice nobody will use them because they will be given persuasive reasons for staying on the bed? How would you broach the issues of making choices if you work with people whose attitude is similar to that of a doctor who said publicly, 'A good patient is one who listens to what I say, believes what I say, accepts what I say and does what I say . . .'?

The antenatal teacher may find herself (either through choice or in response to pressure) teaching to maintain the status quo. Some teachers argue that it is more sensible to prepare parents to accept without question the management that they are likely to receive. Not to do so can lead to difficulties with colleagues, managers and obstetricians. Raising parents' awareness can also mean that they come back after the birth, feeling disappointed and upset because their experience fell short of their expectations.

However, teaching for compliance denies parents the information they deserve and the opportunity to make choices for themselves and their babies. It turns them into passive recipients of care, encouraging dependence and reliance on experts at the expense of developing confidence in the innate ability of a woman's body to nurture her baby, give birth and then, together with her partner or on her own, function as a responsible parent.

Teaching in a way that empowers parents to make their own choices and state their own wishes when the system overtly or tacitly demands compliance, requires skill and some courage. The teacher may appear disloyal – even subversive – and it requires tact, patience and skill to find approaches which are effective and do not rock the boat too drastically. We explore this issue in more detail in Chapter 20.

Teaching for choice

The approach we favour puts the parents at the centre. We try to run a course in which expectant parents participate in choosing the topics to be covered. The teacher aims to identify and meet *their* needs and to create a learning environment that enables people to talk about what really matters to *them*. It offers parents the information and skills that *they* see as relevant.

Parent-centred classes take account of what people already know, of individual needs and concerns, and encourage participants to learn from and to support each other. When teaching for choice, balanced information is crucial because what's right for one person will not be right for another. Flexibility is essential because everybody is different and no two labours are the same. The end result will not be conformity, but will enable each to choose what seems best for them in the specific situation that they are facing.

In conclusion

Antenatal classes can reinforce the parents' passivity, acceptance and dependence on 'experts'. They can be used to encourage compliance with hospital routines and procedures. They can give people a set of instructions to follow or they can contain forceful or over-simplistic advice about health issues.

Alternatively, antenatal classes can build self-confidence by encouraging people to build on their own knowledge, to question and evaluate. They can help people to be flexible and work out their own solutions. They can enable prospective parents to see themselves as competent and able to make informed choices for themselves and for their baby – something that is automatically expected of them by society from the time they take their baby home till the child is grown up.

It is because we believe that parent-centred classes are the most effective and the most fun for both parents and teachers that we wrote this book. As you read, there may be times when you feel that, however much you want to, it would be quite impossible to work in some of the ways we suggest. We realize that resources and the scope for change are often limited. You may be teaching classes in difficult circumstances and be under a variety of constraints. If so, you may not be able to make the changes you want to overnight. It may take time and patience to achieve your goals.

We make no apology for being idealistic and setting out the very best we know, for without a vision nothing great is likely to be achieved.

Further reading

The International Standard Book Number (ISBN) is given where possible and should be quoted when ordering the book from your bookseller.

Buzan, Tony (1981) *Make the Most of Your Mind,* Pan, London (ISBN 0-330-26230-0).

Enkin, Murray, Keirse, Marc and Chalmers, Iain (1989) *A Guide to Effective Care in Pregnancy and Childbirth,* Oxford University Press, Oxford (ISBN 0-19-261916-0).

Rogers, Carl (1983) *Freedom to Learn for the 80s,* Charles Merrill, Ohio, USA (ISBN 0675-200121-07).

Rogers, Jennifer (1989) *Adults Learning,* Open University Press, Milton Keynes (ISBN 0-335-09215-2).

Part II

The basics of an antenatal course

5

Planning a course

This chapter describes one way of developing a course plan that will encourage active participation and be flexible enough to adapt to the needs expressed by the people you teach. It leaves to you the choice of topics and the order in which they are covered. So, although your course may be similar to others, the final product will be based on your own careful thinking and planning.

If you want to design a course or review what you already do, you could work through the suggestions in this chapter on your own or, alternatively, you could invite several colleagues to work with you. Either way, you will need four or five hours of uninterrupted time and (if you work in a group) plenty of open communication, respectful listening and negotiation.

Preliminary questions

Who are you designing the course for? Take a moment to consider the questions shown in the box overleaf.

An open or a closed group?

Before you start to plan, decide what kind of group you want to teach. Will it be an open or closed one?

Open groups

An open group is one which accepts anyone who arrives and which becomes a new entity at every session. Several ways of forming open classes exist. Perhaps you will offer a series of classes with a different theme each week. People can join the cycle at any point, leaving when their baby arrives or when they feel they have had enough. In other open groups, parents are encouraged to wait and join at the beginning of the cycle. The group remains an open one if there is no system for discovering who will come and no commitment from individuals to attend all or most of the course. Participants opt in or out at will.

Open groups offer advantages and disadvantages to both parents and teachers.

- Is it for women only? If so, are there sessions for fathers? How many?
- Is your course for women and their partners? Are labour companions invited? Or the mother's mother?
- Is the course primarily for first-time mothers with second-timers free to come along if they wish? Or do you cater exclusively for primips? Do you make time for the special needs of multiparity by offering women with more than one child their own class or gearing certain sessions to their needs.
- Is the course for women in the last third of their pregnancy, or can they start at any time they wish? Or is there an 'earlybirds' class for those less than 16 weeks pregnant?

Advantages for parents in open groups

- Maximum flexibility as to starting dates.
- If the cycle is continuous, there's a chance to catch a particular topic the next time it comes around.
- The format suits those who find it hard to plan ahead.
- A minimum commitment encourages those who might be daunted by a whole course to give a single session a try.
- The more detached, formal style of open groups may appeal to people who are unused to interactive groupwork or worried about what might be asked of them.

Disadvantages for parents in open groups

- The group functions more as an audience with a teacher rather than as a group with a leader, so most of the benefits of groupwork are lost.

- Individuals find it hard to get to know each other, so relationships within the group do not change from week to week.
- Emotive topics which allow parents to express and share strong feelings are difficult or impossible to raise.
- Parents can encounter topics in illogical sequences – say, safety in the home, followed by immunization, followed by early pregnancy then the hospital tour.

Advantages for teachers in open groups

- There is less administration, fewer letters to write and only minimal booking arrangements to operate.
- You stand a better chance of enticing people who are reluctant to attend a whole course to try one session.
- You have greater scope for a rotating schedule of teachers, covering holidays, sickness, etc.

Disadvantages for teachers in open groups

- Because it is difficult to get to know class members, there is less chance of ensuring that each participant has access to the information and the skills she or he might need.
- There is little scope for using many group skills yet the skills that *are* useful require high levels of experience in groupwork. For example, the teacher will need to adapt her programme to deal with any number of people at a moment's notice; she will need to know how to turn strangers into participants within minutes. Most teachers learned these skills by working with groups and may find it frustrating to be working with an ever-changing audience.
- There is pressure on the teacher to take centre stage and hold the session together – something inexperienced teachers find particularly difficult.

Closed groups

Instead of an open group, you could decide to run a group where everyone knows from the first meeting who will be a member of the group and where participants have a certain degree of commitment to attending the group. Even closed groups have changes, of course. For example, people may successfully join the group on the second meeting if the class knows in advance that another member is expected. (After the second week, joining becomes more difficult since the group has begun to establish its own unique identity and ground rules.) Alternatively, group members may drop out after a few sessions because they decide that the course is not for them or because unexpected obstetric events intervene. Despite these changes, the group remains fairly constant because even those not actually present continue to be regarded as members of the group.

Closed groups have a different character from open groups and, like them, will also have both advantages and disadvantages.

Advantages for parents in closed groups

- The class has time to develop as a group, with all the benefits that brings.
- The group can set its own agenda.
- As trust grows, members can address riskier or more emotive issues.
- Group members are often at roughly the same point in their pregnancies.
- Everyone starts together with a logical flow of topics following over several weeks.

Disadvantages for parents in closed groups

- Many may be excluded if a limit is set on the number of people in the group.
- In order to secure a place on a limited entry group, parents need to be well informed and able to plan ahead.
- A substantial commitment is needed as to time and availability. This presumes parents have a suitably settled lifestyle and the ability to predict what they will be doing for several weeks ahead.
- Some parents are uncomfortable with groupwork and unwilling to participate actively, preferring the more passive role of audience.

Advantages for teachers in closed groups

- You have a wider range of options as to what you can comfortably do with a settled group.
- You can see group members changing and developing.
- You can give the group time to do things at their own pace.
- You can adapt the course to meet the particular needs of the group.

Disadvantages for teachers in closed groups

- You will probably have to organize and run a booking system.
- You will probably have to limit numbers and will thus be unable to offer classes to everyone who wants them.
- You are unlikely to attract people who are usually seen as the most in need of classes, reaching instead those who are motivated, articulate and well informed about local services.

Making the choice

Weighing up the pros and cons like this may help you decide which kind of classes you think will be best for you and for parents. However, the choice may not be what suits you, but whether it is best to go for quality or quantity. Some teachers feel obliged to welcome everyone who might want classes and thus, they argue, they can only run open groups. Others interpret their responsibility as an antenatal teacher differently. They argue that it makes no sense to judge effectiveness just by totting up the number of people who pass through your classes if nothing significant happens to them along the way. A closed group, they believe, stands the best chance of helping parents to learn, to change and to make friendships that will be of mutual benefit postnatally. Organizing a booking system isn't really all that difficult once you decide the benefits to parents are worth the effort and are convinced that this kind of group makes the most effective use of the teacher's precious time and energy.

Of course, there is also a middle way. Some teachers offer a package of classes which make up a course, accept all who come and then try to give those present an experience that brings them back for more. Without the formalities of booking and commitment, they nevertheless find that, in time, the group is relatively stable.

How will you resolve the question of whether closed, semi-closed or open classes are best for you and the parents you teach?

Deciding what topics to cover

Begin by asking yourself the three questions in the box overleaf. Your answers to these three questions will produce three lists. In the first list you will find the *information* you could include in an antenatal course. The second list will have all the *physical skills* – things parents can do with their bodies – that you want parents to master through attending your course. And the last list will have *attitudes and feelings* that expectant parents commonly experience and could benefit from exploring and discussing together.

- What do parents need to know to cope well with the changes of pregnancy, the challenges of giving birth and the first few days of parenthood?
- What do parents need to learn to do with their bodies in order to feel as confident and comfortable as possible through the rest of their pregnancy, when giving birth, and when they are caring for their new baby?
- What attitudes and feelings would parents benefit from discussing and exploring with others to understand better what they have already experienced in pregnancy and to prepare for the birth and the early weeks of parenthood?

It may take some time to list the topics you think belong under these headings. If you are working in a group, encourage people to begin by brainstorming. This means that everyone calls out their ideas quickly and without censoring. These are all charted, and discussion and debate are postponed until the flow of ideas has stopped.

Table 5.1 Possible subheadings for the topic 'breastfeeding'

Information	*Physical skills*	*Attitudes/feelings*
What's in breastmilk	Holding the baby	Do I want to?
How a 'letdown' works	Positioning baby at breast	Who thinks I should or shouldn't?
What's colostrum	Encouraging a wide mouth	'Failure'
What's a good latch	Latching baby on	Feeding in public
Consequences of poor latch	Breaking suction	Sex, sexy feelings
Supply and demand	Eliciting reflexes	Asking for help
Physiology of the breast	Recognizing swallowing	
Reflexes		
Where to get help		
As a contraceptive		

Brainstorming is also a good way of working if you are by yourself. It encourages free thinking which you can refine later. Your list, like that produced by each individual or group that tackles this task, will be unique.

It may take a while to get used to thinking of topics under these three headings. You may find that most of your early efforts contain elements from all three kinds of activities. For example, 'breastfeeding' will have the possible sub-headings shown in Table 5.1.

In all your lists, make sure you include only the appropriate topics, or elements of a topic, under each of the three headings.

Within the box are a few suggestions about what information you might cover in an antenatal course. Use, discard, change and adapt this list to get your own thinking going. Include in your own 'information' list only the things you want them to know. Make sure the topics you list are relevant to the people you teach. When appropriate, include information particularly relevant to men, grandmothers or labour supporters.

Information

Physical changes in pregnancy
Diet
Fetal development
What is a contraction?
Stages of labour
What to take to hospital
Monitoring
Episiotomy
Forceps
Normal newborn behaviour
Breastfeeding
What's on co-op cards
Stillbirth and handicap – what happens?
Role of the health visitor/ midwife
Hormonal changes in pregnancy
Dental care
Hazards to baby in pregnancy
How labour starts
Going to hospital
Induction
Pain relief
What happens during a CS
Symptoms of PN depression
Usual hospital routines
Bottle feeding

Now go back to the questions on page 32 and generate two more lists. In the next two boxes are some more suggestions to get you started.

Physical skills

Pelvic floor exercises
Pelvic rocking/tilting
Posture
Relaxation in pregnancy/labour/postnatally
Easing backache in pregnancy
Easing backache in labour
Perineal massage
Positioning a breastfeeding baby
Latching on a breastfeeding baby
Looking and sounding assertive
Breathing awareness
Breathing for first stage
Breathing for second stage
Positions for first stage
Positions for second stage
Coping with a caesarian
Massage
Bathing a baby
Changing nappies
Comforting a crying newborn
Mixing a bottle
Positioning and feeding a bottlefed baby

Attitudes and feelings

Changes in financial situation
Changes in couple's relationship
Feelings about the woman's changing body
Changes in sex life in pregnancy/postnatally
New ways of organising the day
Fears/hopes to do with pregnancy
Fears/hopes to do with labour
Fears/hopes to do with new parenthood
Feelings about pain
Woman's new self-image in pregnancy/motherhood
New friendships
Fears about stillbirth and handicap
Feelings about feeding
Disappointment and 'failure' should hopes not materialize
Fitting the new baby into the family
What new fathers need
Stresses of new fatherhood
Relationships with medical people and care team
What's a good father/mother?

Selecting priority topics

You will only have the time to cover a few topics thoroughly in your course, no matter how long it will be. So first, ask yourself *for each item on your three lists*:

- Can parents get this elsewhere? For example, is this information given as a routine part of antenatal care? Can I reasonably expect the postnatal ward midwives to cover this?
- Do parents *need* to know this? Or do this? Or think about this?
- What would be the effects of *not* including this in the course?

On these grounds you might eliminate dental care or diet, perineal massage or a discussion of parents' finances from your course plan. None of these things is a trivial matter, but given the limited time available you must choose. Stick to what you see as needs and let the parents add their own wants. As a rough guide, allow no more than 20 topics per list for a six-week course, less for a shorter one and more for a longer one. If you have more than this number, you won't be able to take the next step in planning your course.

Laying out your course plan

The next task is to allocate individual topics to particular sessions. You can do this by creating different coloured cards, one colour for each of the lists. For example, you could write all the information topics, one by one, on blue cards, physical skills on, say, yellow cards and all the attitude topics could go onto pink ones producing a multi-coloured pack of topics.

Next, make white number cards, one number for each session that you plan to include in your course. Say you plan to teach six classes with one fathers' evening, you would make cards numbered 1 to 6, plus one white card labelled 'Fathers'.

Now you are ready to assemble your course.

- First, place the numbered cards in a line, across the floor in front of you. Each white number card denotes an individual class in your course.
- Hand out the cards to the group or work through them yourself.
- Place each card under the number denoting the class where you think that topic best fits. For example, you might put 'How labour

starts' under the number 2, showing that you plan to do it in the second class and place a card with 'Positions for second stage' under the number 4 showing it will come in the fourth class.

- Keep placing the cards under the appropriate class number and move them as your ideas change.
- Make duplicates for topics that will be covered more than once.
- If you are working in a group, take time to discuss your decisions and negotiate between members of the group as you establish the best spot for certain cards. Here is one way to begin laying out the cards. We have used dots and stripes to indicate different colours.

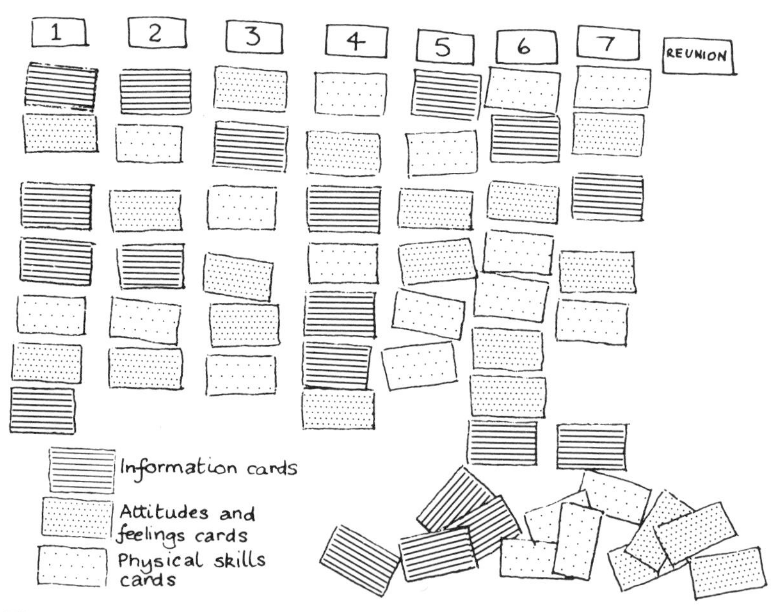

Figure 5.1

Fine-tuning your course plan

When all the cards are in place, start weeding. Each topic will take at least 10 minutes to do *well*. Of course you could just say something about it in less time, but remember what was already said about adult learning. In order for parents to understand and remember whatever you teach, you have to allow time for questions, discussions, practice and problem-solving. A few topics will take a good deal longer than

10 minutes. So in a one-hour class you will only have room for four or possibly five topics if you want to leave time for the group to settle, for people to talk and catch up with each other's news and for the unexpected events which always occur. In a two-hour class, you might handle eight or nine cards. The rest must go.

It is often hard to discard topics. You may feel tempted to sneak them back by amalgamating several under headings ('Let's see . . . forceps, monitoring and induction – oh, I'll call that "interventions" . . .'). Or you might keep a long list of cards in one class saying, 'Oh, I'll just spend a minute or so on each.' However, you will serve parents better if you cover a few things well than if you dash through a dozen superficially. Besides, you could never cover *everything* even if you had all the time in the world.

Now stand back and look at the colours rather than the words on each card. Is any class top-heavy with one colour? The best sessions offer a mixture of all three activities – taking in information, practising skills, and discussing or sharing ideas and feelings among the group. Keep moving the cards until each session contains a balance of all three activities.

Then check that topics are covered in a logical order and that there is a natural flow of material throughout the course. Does your plan reflect the way in which parents are likely to encounter the events of pregnancy, labour, birth and parenting?

Finally, look within each session, viewing each column of cards as a chronological record of the class. The best sessions offer the group a new kind of activity every 10 minutes or so. So, for example, if you start with information-giving, have you followed it with a card for physical skills or one for discussion? And after a discussion, is the next card a change of pace? You should see a variety of colours as you move down the line – do you?

Recording your course plan

After all this checking and moving cards about, you should be left with a patchwork grid containing the key topics and activities you want to include in your course in the order in which you think they are best presented to parents. By writing down your plan, you create a permanent record of your thinking.

Another way of recording your plan is to mark each card to show the number of the class and the order in which you plan to tackle it (for instance 3–3 might mean the third item in Class 3). You could then store your cards in individual envelopes, one for each session. This method allows you to tailor each course to fit the group, moving cards between envelopes to reflect what actually happened, then re-ordering the pack at the end of the course. For example, if they want to cover the third stage in the first class but you'd planned to do this in the sixth, you can respond to what the group wants then afterwards, retrieve the 'third stage' card from Week 6 or whenever *you* planned to do it and put it in the envelope for Class 1. You can also re-file cards for planned topics that weren't covered and, in that way, remind yourself to cover them later. Then, at the end of the course, replace the cards in their original place for next time.

In conclusion

Building a course using colour-coded cards offers several benefits. The cards-in-envelopes system is a boon for people who share classes because each teacher can pick up the pack for that week and see at a glance what needs to be done and pass on updated information to the next person. By taking large topics apart and converting them to cards, you put some order into your own ideas and have a tangible way of finding out what others are thinking without getting bogged down in personalities and hobby-horses. Most importantly, in the course that results, you jumble up listening and doing, discussing and looking, talking and trying things out so you keep people awake, involved and learning.

If you have read straight through this chapter and now feel it all sounds much too complicated, try it. You'll find it allows you to convert a swirling mass of ideas and a blank sheet of paper into a coherent and highly personal course plan.

6

Getting started

Publicizing your group

Some antenatal teachers have to work quite hard to publicize their classes and to establish a reputation among childbearing women. Others have a steady stream of people wanting to join. So long as pregnant women are telling others that your classes are interesting and fun, you will not need to put effort into publicity. On the other hand, in order to become established or if you wish to widen the 'net', bringing in different groups of people, then you may need to give some thought to publicity.

One obvious route is to use existing points of contact between pregnant women and health professionals. They meet at clinics, GP surgeries, hospital booking clinics and other places where staff might discuss classes, put up a poster, pass on a booklet or deliver a letter about classes to each woman. By using this approach, you reach most pregnant women with information *in writing* which they can refer to later.

Organizing the handouts or designing the posters takes time but once done you need only top up stock or reassess their effectiveness. However, standardized written material can feel impersonal and converts few who are reluctant or unsure about the whole business of classes.

There are ways to mitigate the disadvantages of relying on printed material. One is to encourage whoever gives it out to offer the receiver time to ask questions, air her own views and think out loud about the issues that might keep her from attending.

Another is to offer handouts that go beyond the necessary data about classes (when, where, who runs them, etc.) and include a sense of expectation and invitation. Could yours do with a facelift? Desk-top publishing techniques offer everyone the chance to produce cheap and cheerful handouts that look professional. If you are not sure how to start, try your local technical college where students are always needing good projects or think through the people who have recently attended your classes. Would one of them have the expertise to get you going?

When you have a first draft of a publicity leaflet, stand back and ask questions like the ones in the box. Your leaflet or publicity material may be the only contact you have with prospective parents before they arrive at your first class, so make sure that written material includes all the information they need to find you with a minimum of trouble. A clear map is usually essential and they may welcome suggestions about public transport, notification of any special signposting, and forewarning of any access difficulties. Will you invite those with disabilities to make their needs known? Include suggestions on what clothes would be appropriate and and one or two sentences on what to expect on the first meeting.

- Does my handout use large print and include plenty of white space?
- Have I used as few words as possible? Which ones could I do without? Are they everyday words or has medical language crept in?
- Are the sentences short?
- Are the words addressed directly to the reader ('you are welcome' rather than 'women are welcome')?
- If men and women are invited, does every single word apply to both sexes?
- Have I used drawings, boxes and lists to break up the text?
- You might even ask yourself, 'Suppose this was an invitation to a party, would I go? Does it sound interesting enough to stir me into making the effort . . . ?'

The venue

The ideal teaching room is well lit, well ventilated, square, private, carpeted and with plenty of storage places. Sadly, most of us have to cope with something far short of this.

Take time to make what you have the best possible place for groupwork. Arrange the chairs so that everyone can see everyone else. If you can, have similar chairs for everyone, make the circle as round as possible, remove any tables or equipment from the middle, and include your chair in the circle. You will find as you work that when people return to a circle from smaller groups, they leave gaps or form a horseshoe shape around you as the teacher. If this happens, encourage them to 'smooth' the circle before you start a discussion or activity (Figure 6.1).

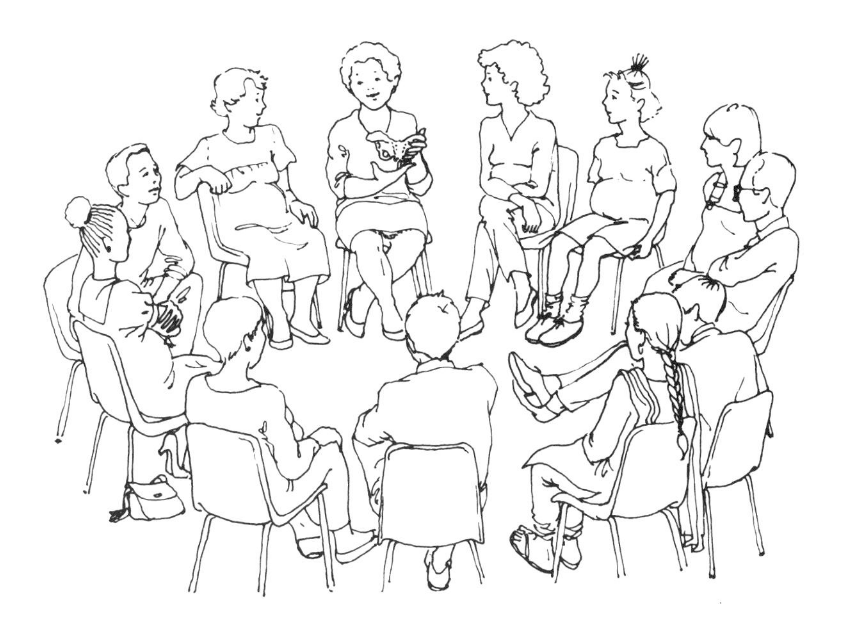

Figure 6.1

If the circle is small in relation to the size of the room, place it near one corner. If the room will not accommodate everyone in one large circle, try two circles, one inside another and move people often, as most do not like sitting in the inside circle surrounded by the larger one. Another way to accommodate many people is to ask couples to double up (him sitting on a cushion between her legs). That will fit more people into a circle, but if you divide them into smaller groups you will have to keep couples together or the men will have no clear place to sit.

The first meeting

People are always apprehensive when they first come to a class, perhaps asking themselves: 'Will I find it?' 'Who else will be there?' 'What will the teacher be like?' or 'What will happen?' Nor is the apprehension one-sided. You might be wondering: 'Who's coming? How many? What will they want? Will this group go well?', and a host of other thoughts. Anxious first-time arrivers often appreciate temporary signs or arrows guiding them from the main front door to wherever you are teaching. When we start a group, we stand at the room door, greet each new arrival, and invite her or him in. That way, we reassure them and ourselves!

For the first week or two in a closed group (and every week in an open one) give some thought to the moments between arrival and the formal start of the class. Can you find ways to keep people from sitting in awkward silence? How about:

- Offering the first arrivals sticky-label name tags and suggesting they write their own names in large letters and then pass on these instructions to the next person who comes in. Organizing this often gets them talking.
- Putting the kettle on and suggesting that people make themselves a drink (put up a sign asking for donations if this is appropriate).
- Mounting a dozen or so photographs on one theme – going to hospital in labour; sleeping newborns; a delivery room – then strewing them on the floor in the centre of the room along with a card containing a large, printed question (e.g. 'What do these make you think of?' 'What's your first thought when you see this?'). New arrivals can be directed to these.
- Spreading out a collection of baby things on the floor, including some you feel are unnecessary, with a card that says, 'Which would *you* collect to be ready for your baby?'
- Putting out library books if this service is offered.

The moment to begin

People are never all present by the appointed starting time and with an open group you never know how many are coming anyway. However, if you wait too long for stragglers, you will find that the number of latecomers goes up week by week. Delaying also disregards the effort made by you and the rest of the group to arrive on time. The best solution is usually to start on time and design the first part of your session in such a way as to allow late-comers to slip into the group with the minimum of fuss. One way is suggested in the next section. Your punctuality will be more effective if it is included when you set the ground rules (see below).

Getting started as a group

From the first moment people start working together as a group, an effective teacher has to keep two strands alive in order for the group to flourish. One strand is called 'the task' and consists of the work that individual members of the group have come together to do. In this case, the task is usually getting ready for the birth of a baby and the early weeks of parenthood. The other strand, called 'the group process', refers to anything the group does to keep them functioning well as a *group*. When your class first meets, they are a room full of individuals that just happen to be in the same place at the same time. If you want them to become a group, you will first have to devote time and energy to getting the process started. Then, during the course, you will need to keep going back to the needs of the group as a *group* to keep it working well.

For some people, suggesting that the group spends time getting acquainted or telling each other about their journey to get there seems a waste of time: 'Why not just get on with it . . . That's why they came!' Those who plunge straight in to work are like housebuilders who start bricklaying ('the task') without spending time drawing up plans and laying the foundations ('the group process'). For a while, just laying bricks seems more efficient, but it soon becomes clear that foundations are essential and for bigger, better, more complex houses, scaffolding is also needed alongside bricklaying. Each of these components – both the task and the 'scaffolding' – will get sometimes more and sometimes less attention as seems appropriate.

The same principles hold true for antenatal groups. The skill comes in judging how much time and attention to devote to the work that parents came together to do and how much to nourishing and assessing the group process. When either is neglected, group members will probably feel frustrated and dissatisfied. Starting the whole business with the group process, by allowing people time to settle, to know each other and to measure how willing they are to contribute, is an investment for later hard work.

People often start slowly and sometimes reluctantly to join the group. For a while they may be shy, unsure of what to do, suspicious or even contrary. If they are treated with gentle respect, given easy, non-threatening things to do, and told exactly what you want of them, they begin to relax and trust both you and each other. After you have started a few groups, you will know that you just have to accept the group's awkwardness until they begin to relate to each other and settle into the work the group is there to do. Two ideas help us feel confident through those sticky early times : the experience that people usually *do* settle, plus a firm conviction that the benefits of working with a group rather than with a passive audience make the effort worth while. These might help you if this is a new way of working.

One way to get started

You could try the following pattern of moves, adapting it to fit the numbers you have. The key points here are to keep pairs together and to move from very small groups to slightly larger ones.

- Talk only for two or three minutes on domestic matters, such as where the fire escape is, how to find the toilets, or when the coffee breaks will be. Then ask them to find someone in the room they don't know. This always makes people rather anxious, so you need to make the task as simple as possible. Tell them how long they will have ('Take 2 minutes each. I will call time in the middle to give you equal time'). Tell them *exactly* what they are to do. For example: 'Tell the other person your name, when your baby is due, and one thing about yourself that has nothing whatsoever to do with babies that you would be willing to share with the whole group. You will not have to tell the other person's name to the rest of the group.'

  Then suggest they stand and move about to find someone to talk with. Stand up yourself to get them going, then check that pairs have formed. If there's an odd number, form a trio and tell them they will take a bit longer but will catch up on the next move. Once they are in pairs, repeat the instruction which they have probably forgotten while they were concentrating on finding a partner.
- Once each person in a pair has had sufficient time, move the pairs into groups of four (leaving any threesome as they are) and

encourage people to move their chairs into a small circle. Ask them to exchange names and due dates and then deal with a particular open question. You could ask, 'Why have you come to these classes?', 'What do you hope to get out of these classes?', or 'What do you hope *won't* happen in these classes?' We usually suggest that no one speaks twice until everyone has spoken once, as a way of encouraging the talkative ones to hold back a bit.

- After five or six minutes, you may hear the noise level drop or see people leaning back and looking less interested. That's a cue to move them on by combining two fours to make groups of eight. Remind them to exchange names and offer them large sheets of paper to list all their reasons for coming, or their hopes and fears for the course. Encourage them to write down the actual words they say, not trying to summarize or dress up ideas in more academic terminology. This takes eight or ten minutes.
- Then bring the whole group back together again. You could follow this with a name round (see below). Where you have more than 16 people, you might acknowledge the difficulty of learning names, rely on name tags, and keep reminding smaller groups to start by exchanging names.

This whole sequence takes about 25 minutes. Whether or not you wish to spend time in this way will depend on how well you want the group to know each other. If they are only meeting for an hour and will not meet again, the foursomes could agree on and list three things they want to do in that time and display their lists on the wall. The whole group could then discuss the lists together. This would take about 25% of your time, but it would be time well spent. Not only would you find out for sure that you were doing what they wanted, but they would be in the mood to talk and interact. You can draw on this for the rest of that hour.

On the other hand, if the group is scheduled to meet several times over the next few weeks, you could decide to spend even more than 25 minutes on helping everyone to meet, talk and set an agenda (see page 50), and you would certainly want to do a name round.

Learning names

Even if people wear name tags, encourage everyone to say her or his name to the whole group. This lets everyone know how each name is pronounced and may encourage the quiet ones, having spoken once, to try speaking again. You might want to negotiate with the group as to what form of address will be used. Will everyone – including the teacher – use first names? Or will everyone have a title (Sister, Miss, Begum, etc.)? If you are working with members of ethnic minority groups, have you discovered how their naming system works so as to be sure you are asking the right questions? You could either do this in advance by consulting a specialist book (see Further Reading at the end of Part II) or do it with the group, asking them for help. It is worth spending time on details of naming, as a group will work better if everyone adopts the same form of address and feels comfortable with it.

Name rounds come in all sorts of styles; for example:

- Say your name.
- Say your name and one thing about yourself. You model this by starting it off. At the first meeting, keep it light and safe ('I'm Judy and I'm wearing blue socks' or 'I'm Judith and I am not sure what colour to paint my bedroom').
- Say your name and something about it.
- Say your name and an adjective that starts with the same letter (Sassy Sally, Round Rachel). This makes people laugh and can be intriguing if you pay attention.
- Pass round a large piece of paper and felt-tip pen and ask everyone to write their name while saying something about it.
- Say your name and share something good about your week.

When you are leading a name round, start with yourself to set the tone, then turn towards each person as they speak. A nod, smile or 'Thank you, Mary' will acknowledge the speaker, but only do so if you actually *are* grateful. People spot false gratitude a mile off! If you set up a round, it is important that you do not let anyone interrupt it. Stories and discussion can wait until everyone has had equal time. You will need to repeat name-learning exercises a surprising number of times if you want expectant parents to learn names. They are so absorbed in their own worlds, or forgetful and anxious, that it takes them longer to fix other people's names in their brains. Groups will welcome a new variant of a name round each time you do it.

As well as rounds, there are name games that some people like; for example:

- Call someone's name while throwing her or him a cushion. Encourage people to ask the names of those they don't know before throwing to them. Some groups hate this, others find that the laughter and movement loosens them and their tongues. In general, you can take calculated risks and not face serious consequences if you allow the group time to react and feed back how they felt about it. Afterwards ask, 'Any reactions. . . . Good? Bad? What was it like?'

- A variation on the cushion throwing is to throw a ball of string, calling names until it is used up, then repeating them as you wind it up.
- The group members arrange themselves in a line alphabetically by first names.
- Play 'My Grandmother went to market and took . . .', where the first person says her name, the next repeats it and adds hers and so on until the grandmother 'takes' everyone in the group. You need to recognize that this makes some people acutely nervous. It will help if the teacher (who should always be last . . . the hardest spot) prompts the early ones to establish that 'cheating ' is acceptable. This game is best done on the second or third meeting.

When the group no longer needs a name round, you might still start the session with a similar exercise. They might each say a good and bad thing that happened in the past week, something new they learned about their baby, or anything else that settles them and allows each person a bit of time and attention from the rest of the group. You could also give them a few minutes to talk in pairs about what happened on their journey to class that day as this is often eventful and prevents people from concentrating on what is happening in the group until it is shared and acknowledged. In all these settling exercises, make sure that you as the teacher join in when you can.

Forming subgroups

The larger your group, the more possibilities you have for subdividing it. A group of about 50 could form:

two groups of 25;
three groups of 18 or so;
four groups of 12 or so;
five groups of 10;
six groups of 8 or 9;

eight or nine groups of 6 or 7;
ten groups of 5;
twelve groups of 4;
eighteen groups of 3;
and 25 pairs.

The combinations are numerous and so, too, are the kinds of activities these sized subgroups can do together. With practice, you will be able to judge which tasks fit best with which sized subgroup. Most groups with more than 14 members function like an audience. You can do some things – brainstorming, showing a video, or delivering a short lecture all work well with this size group – but you will need smaller groupings for other activities.

In general, people are more likely to feel safe to talk openly in twos or groups of three or four. These are good combinations for discussing emotive topics or helping the quieter people to talk. People in groups of five or six can share experiences, especially if they have already had practice listening to each other in twos and threes. Seven to nine people can generate ideas and make lists ('All the good things about *x*'). Fewer than this many people in a group might not have enough information between them to successfully complete a task that requires a certain amount of knowledge. You must make absolutely sure that whatever you ask of them, they will be able to do it.

Here are some ways we divide a class. Choose new techniques often, as it seems to keep people entertained wondering what will come next!

- *In twos*: Check you have an even number, then ask every other person to pair with whoever is on their left.
- *In fours*: Join the two pairs that have worked together. Depending on the size of the group, number '1, 2, 3, 4' etc. round the big group or use a variation like 'orange, apple, pear, banana' etc. or anything else you can think of. You can form threes, fives and sixes this way, too.
- *In half*: Draw the 'equator' through the middle of the group, making sure you vary the division each time. Number '1, 2–1, 2' round the group (or a variation). Ask people to fold their arms or clasp their hands, then divide according to whether they have the left or right thumb/arm on top. Call out birth months (January to July in one group, August to December in another) or initials of their first names. The last three techniques work best with groups of 20 or more.

You can also group people who have something in common, such as men and women; neighbours; people who are cared for by the same team of midwives or consultant; primips; multips; or those at similar stages in pregnancy. These groups can share whatever experiences, information and feelings are particularly relevant to them.

Whenever you are subdividing a group, the division goes more smoothly if you:

- Ensure people know their number/name before anyone moves (say something like, 'Would all the twos raise your hand . . . and the fours? Everyone clear? . . .').
- Make sure they know where they are going.
- Tell them how long they will be working together.
- Give clear instructions as to what you want them to do. Write it on a flipchart or board or hand round a card to each group.
- Tell people if there will be any reporting back to the big group.

The more people there are, the longer it will take for subgroups to form. However, moving is useful as it allows people to chat, stretch, and recharge their batteries. After the small groups have finished their time together, allow time for everyone to return to their original spot if they wish.

Setting the contract

All groups develop patterns of interaction even if they are not acknowledged. The sooner your group establishes ground rules and agrees to share responsibility in maintaining them, the better it will function. You might propose some rules yourself, write them down, ask for any more that the group want added then display them for all to see. Below are some we use.

Confidentiality

By this, we mean not only that people agree that what is said or done in this group stays in the room, but that what people say or do in small groups stays there, too. People are often willing to say things to three or four that they would be horrified to hear repeated in a group of 16. This constraint includes prompting along the lines of, 'That's like what you were saying, Maureen, when we talked about . . .'.

Equal time

Suggest that everyone pays attention to how often and how long they speak. This will help the talkers hold back and listen. Given time and space, the reluctant ones *will* offer their ideas and experiences. By agreeing to share time equally (or thereabouts), the group takes responsibility for carrying it out, although they will need frequent prompts in the early sessions lest the dominant people fall back on old habits.

Listening with respect

We all find it easier to listen to those we agree with than to those with whom we disagree. By suggesting they listen as hard to the differences between them as to the similarities, you help people feel freer to speak and you encourage those who are firmly fixed in any one notion to begin to explore other ways of thinking and feeling. This is especially important in the fields of pregnancy and birth, where few issues have a clear right or wrong answer yet most have passionate advocates – and that holds for antenatal teachers, too. Your own tolerance, respect and gentleness will of course set the tone for the rest of the group. Have you acknowledged both sides of most contentious issues as well as deciding where you stand?

Setting an agenda for the course

You are as unlikely to start a course without a plan as you are to start a long journey without a map and itinerary. Unlike most of your group, you have 'travelled' this way before so you are likely to know the topics and activities that are usually relevant and useful. Your general knowledge has to be tailored to suit each group and, since you are not a mind reader, you will only be able to answer questions like, 'What is *really* worrying them? What particular emphasis does this or that person want? How do they want to spend their time?', if you ask them in ways that might trigger a straight answer. Here are a few ways to try:

- Ask them to list topics or hopes and fears in small groups (see page 45), then display the charts, gather people around them and talk through what they have written. Ask questions, add topics, and expand in writing on their charts. Keep the charts, bring them out two or three times during the course and check on what you have and have not covered, crossing out the former and adding the latter. You may need to do one of the prioritizing exercises described below.

- Divide people into groups of five or six, pass out eight or 10 cards similar to those used to plan a course (see Chapter 5), with broad topic headings, and ask them to choose six they wish to cover in the course. If you have only a short time, ask them to choose fewer topics. Then suggest they put the cards in some kind of order reflecting how important they see that topic. They will have to negotiate within the group and, in so doing, you will start a discussion as well as accomplish a task.
- Display a list of topics on the wall and ask everyone to tick the two or three they most want to cover (Figure 6.2). Even in a group of 25, priorities will quickly emerge.

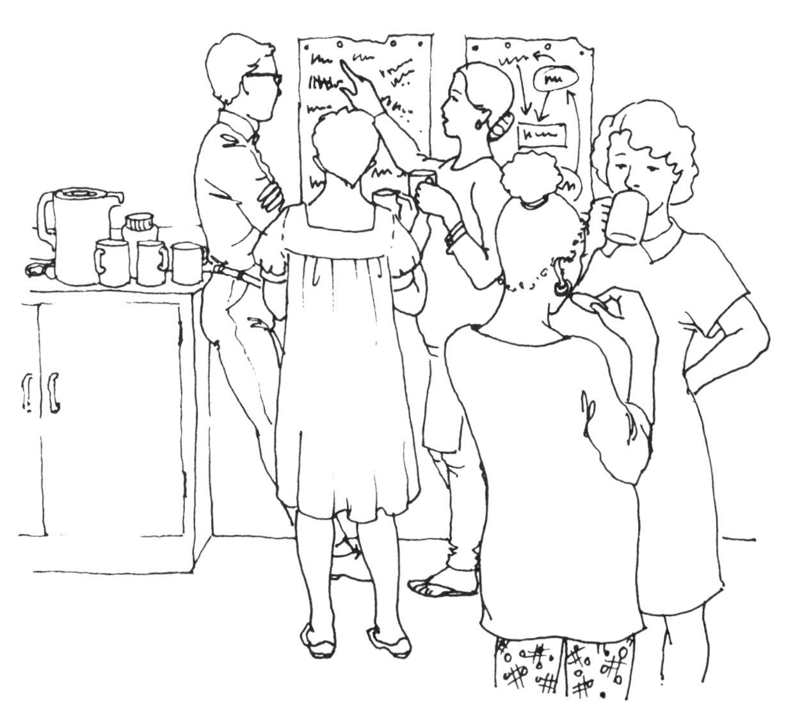

Figure 6.2

- Pass round a suggestion box and slips of paper. Ask everyone to write down the one topic or idea or worry they would feel sad *not* to have covered during the time the group has together. Then make a list of these, do a ticking exercise and plan how to accommodate every one of these central issues before the group finishes.

Implicit in any agenda-planning exercise is your commitment to adapt what you do to accommodate participants' wishes. You not only have to do it, you have to be *seen* to do it. Make time regularly to check if what you are doing is what they *want* to be doing. We repeat these exercises several times during the life of the group. Unless we do, we won't know if what we are doing is the best way for them to spend their time, nor will they feel that the group truly belongs to them.

Taking time and trouble to plan how you welcome people and get your group started means that you will start your course on good foundations. It is a sound investment.

7

Giving information

In many antenatal classes, giving information is the central activity occupying most of each session. Often, this means that the teacher holds the floor for long periods,while the parents sit and listen – or sometimes just sit! Ironically, if you ask either side how they feel about this arrangement, neither is enthusiastic. The teacher may long for more participation and feedback during the session and be genuinely dismayed to discover that little of what she said has been remembered. Some parents will be satisfied with listening to someone giving information, but many will report feeling bored or frustrated during such a session. Many are disconcerted later on, when passive listening has not equipped them to cope with labour or early parenthood.

There is another way, as you may have already discovered. This chapter suggests how you can move towards more effective ways of sharing information. It starts with suggestions on giving an effective lecture, continues with offering other ways to give information then finishes with ways of drawing information from the group. You could use this chapter in isolation, dipping in to find ways of doing what you already do differently. But the ideas and exercises will work better if you have done two other things first:

- Do a bit of rethinking about your job as teacher and about the parents' job as learners in an antenatal class. Chapter 3 describes why experiential learning (i.e. learning based on doing things and using information) is more effective than passive lecture-type learning. Theories of adult learning have led us to rewrite the well known saying, 'Use it or lose it'. We now say, as far as information is concerned, 'Unless you use it, you never had it in the first place'.
- Before thinking about how you give information, reconsider your course plan as suggested in Chapter 5. Unless you do, you could fall

victim to a common trap: information sprawl. Information sharing is only *one* of the things parents and teachers can usefully do in an antenatal class. All too often, so much time is devoted to giving information that there is not enough left for anything else. Planning helps you put information in perspective.

The five-minute lecture and how to give it

You may feel, after reading the last few paragraphs, that a knowledgeable professional has no business talking at all. Perhaps lectures are somehow taboo? Not at all. Lectures continue to be a useful tool for any antenatal teacher. But you owe it to yourself and your listeners to be really effective when giving information. The key points discussed below can help you do this.

Keep it short

How long can you really listen and absorb information? Most of us can only manage 20 minutes and, if we are honest, our attention drops after 10. Pregnancy shortens even this brief span because hormones, anxiety and tiredness all interfere with active listening. As a rule of thumb, pregnant women (and often their partners) can only expend maximum effort to hear, react, process and store information for five minutes.

Prospective parents *seem* to listen for much longer than this, of course. They are often so hungry for information and so anxious to 'get things right' that they will sit quietly for many minutes, but nothing much is happening inside their heads. One way to help parents judge how much energy to put into listening is to tell them before you begin that you intend to talk only for five minutes. This also encourages those who dread lectures not to switch off.

Cover large topics in sections

When you plan your lecture, the first step is to take the topic apart. For instance, labour can be treated as a story with many 'chapters' – how labour starts, changeover to active labour, early first stage, late first stage and so on. Each could be described in about five minutes, with time in between the chapters for some other activity – say, appropriate positions for that stage of labour.

Any topic can be covered in this way. Dissecting 'pain relief' into component parts would produce an ever-widening number of topics under one heading. Some of them are suggested in the boxes, although you could well sub-divide the topic differently.

Pharmacological and non-pharmacological pain relief: examples of each.

What's on offer in our hospital; what's available at home.

Pethidine:
What is it?
How does it feel?
How do I use it?

Entonox:
What is it?
How does it feel?
How do I use it?

Epidural:
What is it?
What does it involve?

Using Pethidine effectively.

Using Entonox effectively.

What an epidural feels like.

Effects of pharmacological pain relief on the baby.

If you give good information for five minutes about each of these boxes, in one two-hour session, you might spend a total of 45 minutes talking to your listening group. So treating information in this way does not necessarily cut down the *total* amount of time you spend giving it, but it does change the style in which you do it. And in the process, you greatly enhance your effectiveness because you increase the chances that people will be actively listening.

Identify essential information

Often, when we introduce the concept of the five-minute lecture to antenatal teachers, they balk at the idea. There is so much to say and it all seems important. It may hurt to leave things out – after all, pregnancy, birth and new parenthood are the things around which your working life revolves. It would be surprising if you didn't find it fascinating and want to share your insights and experience with others. But limited time, limited attention spans and the sheer impossibility of telling the group everything will force cuts on you.

One way to sort out the essential from the fascinating but optional, is to imagine this scene. You are at an airport and your transatlantic flight is about to be called. You are making a long-distance phone call to a close friend who is 8½ months pregnant. Just as your flight is announced, your friend says, 'Tell me about breastfeeding'. You only have time for three short sentences. What do you say?

To breastfeed, she *must* know how to position the baby, how to recognize a good latch and the law of supply and demand. Without these three basics, breastfeeding won't work. Of course, there is more to it – whole libraries of books have been written on breastfeeding! But what does she *have* to know to get started?

Exactly the same scenario will help you decide the three (or four) points that are essential in any topic. What are the three essential things about second stage? Or pain relief? Or postnatal depression? But be careful to give facts. Often when we ask people to come up with their own personal 'three essential points', what they offer are not facts such as:

'Pethidine works in about 20 minutes.'
'Epidurals are put in by anaesthetists.'
'Entonox is a mixture of 50% nitrous oxide and 50% oxygen.'

but feelings or opinions such as:

'You shouldn't feel guilty if you have an epidural.'
'Pethidine babies cry more for the first few months (*sic*).'
'Entonox is a lovely form of pain relief.'

Telling another person how to feel doesn't work. Nor can you assume that the other person shares your beliefs. Facts, on the other hand, are of concrete use to people.

Tell them these three things three times

Once you have dissected your topic into five-minute chunks and decided the few messages you wish to convey, the following pattern of delivery will increase the chances that your facts are heard and absorbed.

- *Tell them what you are going to say.* 'I want to talk about what women say about having forceps; about how you can help yourself; and about the things that might help you afterwards. . . .'
- *Then give the information.* Offer two sentences quoting what women say about forceps . . . one sentence quoting a man's experience. Then two suggestions for coping with forceps during the birth – each of no more than one or two sentences. Then one or two ways of keeping comfortable and speeding recovery.
- End by *summarizing* the key points, using different phrases.

Delivering information in this way takes a bit of practice but the effort expended will be worth it. You could try out your first efforts on a friend or a small group of supportive colleagues. It ought to fit comfortably into a coffee break!

In general, people will only remember a few points, and in five minutes you will only have time to tell them between three and five things. Have you had the experience of offering them many ideas yet their remembering only a few? By treating topics as we suggest, you at least increase the chance that your group goes home with the three key points you *intended* them to remember.

Other ways of giving information

The five-minute lecture is only one of many ways to convey information. What other ways might you use? You might go through all the information topics you plan to cover, asking yourself for each one, 'How else besides my talking about it could they end up with this information?' The rest of this chapter suggests a few ways to answer this question. You will find more about this in Chapters 9 and 10.

Posters and leaflets

You will increase the chances that parents notice and absorb the message if posters are changed regularly. It is easy to tell that a particular poster has been there for ages. As soon as the viewer realizes this, the message loses some of its impact.

Some posters need no words. One parentcraft room we worked in had a collage of dozens and dozens of snapshots of newborn babies, each labelled with his or her name on a small card in the lower left corner: Angela, Gary, Deepak, Catherine, Mercy. That poster's message was, 'We love and value babies . . .'. The collage was unfinished and the empty lower right corner seemed to say, 'And we are waiting for yours . . .'.

Some posters need words. The simpler the written message, the more likely it will be 'heard' and understood. So never use three words when one will do. Use an image instead of a word if you can. Search for colourful turns of phrase. Finally, value white space because it allows the eye to 'think'.

Attractive posters can serve as room brighteners or decoration, but beware of using too many. We have worked in rooms full of posters, even finding several at eye level for the 'captive audience' in the toilet. Stand back and look at your walls. If you came into the room for the first time, would they look friendly and attractive? Or would all these posters look busy, bossy and just too much effort to take in?

Handouts

Many parents like handouts, especially ones created specifically for them. If you make your own, do find a cheap, flexible way of producing them because you are sure to want to improve and update them as time goes by.

Topics that are particularly suited to treatment with handouts include:

- Anything that can be listed:
  - what to take to hospital,

  - hospital visiting times,
  - an A to Z of pain relief (A is for acupuncture, B is for baths, . . . S is for socks, sunshine and shouting! . . .).
- Any step-by-step procedure:
  - mixing a bottle,
  - the postnatal going-home procedures,
  - postnatal exercise routines.
- Any topic where parents might benefit from reviewing before you cover it in the group:
  - pharmacological pain relief,
  - the pros and cons of a birth plan,
  - a selection of possible support a labour companion could offer.
- Any topic that parents often find difficult to grasp:
  - signs of the onset of labour,
  - what signs are and are not serious in a newborn baby.

Drawing out information already present in the group

So far, this chapter has concentrated on how to provide parents with more information. In fact, parents do not come to antenatal classes as empty vessels waiting to be filled with facts. They already have information, although they sometimes need your help to recognize the fact. They may also want to check out with you whether their information is correct. And you will certainly want to assess what they know. You may also wish to reshape the information they come with to resemble something closer to your experience or knowledge. Several techniques may help you do this.

A discussion often provides plenty of information both for other group members and for the teacher. Chapter 9 covers ways of starting and maintaining discussion.

There may be topics you feel sure that many (if not all) of the group will have ideas about already. For example, in 1989, listeriosis (an infection caused by bacteria found in some cooked foods and soft cheeses) was in the news – every pregnant woman knew about this. As well as the current 'hot topic', there will be perennial favourites. Pain relief is regularly covered by popular pregnancy magazines; and everyone will have heard stories about how labour starts. In most groups, the more academic members will have read several books. If you want to find out what they know about a given topic and affirm their knowledge, try a paperchase. Here's how:

- Head two or more large sheets of paper (see page 279 for cheap sources) with a word or question. Suppose you wanted to pool knowledge about caesarian section. One paper might say 'Why it is done'; others might say 'What happens just before the operation?', 'What happens during the operation?', 'What happens just afterwards?', 'Ways to get better' and so on. The number of questions and statements you set will depend on the size of your primary group. Each small group needs five or six members to be sure of having enough information between them to do the task.
- Give them a few minutes to brainstorm and write down, higgledy-piggledy, what they know. Encourage them to add their own questions, too. Then pass the sheet on to another group.
- That group adds their thoughts, answers the questions if they can, and writes down their own questions if any spring to mind.
- After a few passes, collect and display all the sheets and invite everyone to look and comment. If any points that you feel were really vital had been missed, you could fill in the gaps.

Make sure all groups use pens of the same colour, then no one should be put on the spot and everyone can be proud of having so much knowledge.

Reshaping inaccurate information

This can be tricky. One way to lessen the need to reshape information is to make sure you never ask a general question of the whole group for which there could be a wrong answer (see pages 73–76 on asking questions). But you will inevitably be offered ideas and opinions that either are inaccurate or that you feel need to be re-examined.

In the example given above (the 'paperchase'), false information on the sheets of paper is no longer directly connected with the person who wrote it and you could find that a subsequent group has done the querying for you. However, tact and care are needed even in these safer conditions to make sure the group members don't feel threatened or diminished. Here are some ways to approach the issues:

- Affirm every idea you get, even ones that are wrong or contrary to what you believe. Respond with, 'That's interesting . . . I can see why you say that . . .' or 'So your sister feels that is what caused her baby to . . .'. This will tell the other person that you have indeed heard her.

- Avoid saying, 'Yes, but . . .'. instead say, 'Yes, and . . .'
- Be gentle. Once you have affirmed an idea, you can shift blatant inaccuracies by saying, 'Well, it's not *quite* like that, it's more like . . .' or ask others in the group, 'What have you heard? What are your thoughts on this?'.

Using new knowledge

The Chinese have a proverb –

> I hear and I forget;
> I see and I remember;
> I do and I understand.

So far, this chapter has concentrated on getting the best out of the first two maxims. If, as in the case of the five-minute lecture, parents only *hear* something, you have to work hard to counter the ever-present risk of forgetting. If you can add other senses like eyes to see posters or your gestures, or ears to hear a tape recording of a crying baby, or touch to show how a tense muscle feels as it relaxes . . . your message becomes more memorable. The section on visual aids (Chapter 14) suggests ways to do this. But *real* learning changes people. It happens when knowledge becomes a tool they can use later to solve problems, make decisions and evaluate their own experience. Skilful tool use requires practice.

It is a counsel of perfection to suggest that you ask parents to *use* every new bit of information you give during the session in which it is offered – life is never so tidy. But you could aim that way and the effort would encourage you to devise more and more ways to get parents doing other things besides listening. As the proverb reminds us, doing leads to understanding. It also leads to ownership. When you use knowledge, it comes to belong to you, the user, rather than to the 'expert' who first offered it.

What can parents do with new information? The simplest form of activity connected with new information is to get people to review it. After you have spoken for a few minutes or shown a video or demonstrated a skill, suggest they turn to the person next to them and say the one thing they would remember . . . or the point they would like to think about at home . . . or the thing they would tell their partner . . . or the bit they liked least/best or any other phrase you can dream up to start them talking. If you want questions, ask the pairs to join in fours and suggest 'What we would like to hear more about . . .'. We find this a useful variation on 'Any questions?' And if the question comes from a group of four, no single person admits 'ignorance'.

There are several other ways you can help people use the information you give in class. They can organize it, solve problems with it and reach conclusions with it. You will find ways of helping the group do these things in Chapter 10.

8

Communicating effectively

It has been estimated that when someone is talking to us, 20% of the information we gain is from what is said. The other 80% comes from the speaker's body language – the non-verbal cues such as gesture, posture, tone of voice or facial expression.

The verbal message is not only the smallest component, it is also the first to be discounted when the body language contradicts what is being said. Suppose you say, 'I'm so glad to be going home', with a flat voice and drooping posture, your listener will be confused by the two messages you are sending and will probably believe the non-verbal clues that say you are *not* glad rather than the words that say you are.

Becoming aware of your own body language

We seldom have opportunities to see or hear ourselves as others do. Many of us carry a lot of embarrassment about the way we look and sound and we also make assumptions which are often inaccurate. There are various ways you can find out about your clarity and tone of voice, about your posture and facial expressions.

To find out about the non-verbal messages you are sending, you will need to seek help from a sympathetic friend or colleague, ask your group, or arrange for someone to video you in action so that you can see for yourself how you come across. Do you look friendly, alert and interested? Do you sound clear and caring? Do you send out cues that make it easy for others to ask you questions? Do you have any distracting mannerisms? Asking for this kind of information is difficult. Giving it is hard, too. You will need clear rules for discussing such things and considerable trust in whoever is offering you their reactions and observations (see Chapter 21 and 23).

Even though *how* you say things matters rather more than *what* you say, it useful to look at the language that is appropriate in an antenatal class. You can work on developing new ways of using language that engages, entertains and reaches out to people. When you do this, they learn more easily and become more responsive, which in turn helps you to develop new and increasingly effective ways of communicating with them.

Reshaping textbook language

Most antenatal educators learned about pregnancy and birth from books by men and women who try hard to be objective. They do this by literally treating topics as 'objects' – holding them at arm's length and assuming that whatever it is they are describing is separate not only from the author's own experience but also from that of the reader. Here is an example of this objective, analytical style:

> The pelvic floor consists of a layer of muscle and fibrous tissue that extends across the lower part of the bony pelvis from the lower edge of the symphysis pubis to the tip of the sacrum.'

You would never guess from reading this sentence that both the author and the reader are sitting on a pelvic floor of his or her own. Such language may be appropriate in a textbook for professionals, but it is less appropriate in a book written for pregnant women. Yet in many, the style lingers on. Here's a description of the second stage of labour from a book read avidly by pregnant women:

> The force of uterine contractions, together with the expulsive efforts involuntarily produced by the mother when the head reaches the muscular floor, serve to push it gradually and slowly down the vagina to be delivered through the vaginal entrance.

The author uses the third person ('the mother', and 'it' to refer to a baby) and the passive voice ('to be delivered') giving little hint that the reader is likely one day soon to participate in what is being described.

Language like this has no place in an antenatal class. Whatever you talk about – be it anatomy, technology, feelings or experiences – you are dealing with issues that intimately affect the people you are talking with, things that are actually present in the room or are anticipated as possible experiences in the near future. Instead of the pelvic floor description already cited, you might offer them something like this, demonstrating on yourself as you talk:

> If you feel this hard bone at the front of your pelvis . . . feel it? . . . and the bony bit back here where your tail would be if you had one . . . feel it? . . . then imagine a sling of muscles between those two points. . . .

If you look back to the first description, you see the last paragraph offers the same facts; but in this second form, the words reach out to parents, draw them in and entertain them all at the same time.

It may take a considerable amount of awareness and persistence to overcome years of reading books which treat pregnant women as objects to be observed. The key points described below may help.

Make it personal

Talk directly to parents instead of using the third person ('she' or 'a pregnant woman'). When you do, you help people to connect what you are saying to themselves . 'The baby' becomes 'your baby' and 'the perineum' can be claimed by every woman in the room, including a female antenatal teacher. However, take care. If you use the pronoun 'you', it needs to apply to *every single person* in the room. 'Your baby' shuts out anyone expecting twins and 'your labour' won't include those anticipating a caesarian. This fact needs to be acknowledged regularly, and sometimes you need to make a special effort to say 'your baby or your babies' or 'your labour or however your baby is born'.

Even more care with the pronoun 'you' is needed when leading a mixed group of men and women. 'Your baby' includes everyone; 'your uterus' will need qualifying ('if you have one . . .') or you can express the idea in other ways ('where your baby is'). Even one or two uses of the word 'you' that exclude the men in the room will cancel out all your assertions about this class being for them too.

Reflect the parents' point of view

This can be achieved in the words you use. 'A delivery' describes the experience of midwives and doctors; parents and babies experience 'a birth'. Hospitals 'discharge' people but parents 'go home'. How could you describe 'hospital admission' in parent-centred language?

It is sometimes more difficult to stand in parents' shoes when describing topics or giving information. For example, when we ask a group of health professionals to describe the feelings and experiences of the second stage of labour, the most common things they mention are time limits, the various movements of the baby and crowning. They also mention the feelings generated by waiting for the baby's birth, excitement at first sighting the head and the hard work involved for mothers and their helpers. When we ask mothers, very different things emerge. Some mention the things described by professionals, but most describe feelings of stretching, burning; the frustration of two-steps-forward-and-one-step-back pushing; feeling stuck and desperate; and pain. When you consider what *you* say about the second stage, whose experience are you describing – Yours? The father's? The mother's? The baby's? All four are valid, but only the last three are helpful to your group.

Use everyday language

It is amazing how quickly medical people adopt a way of speaking that is quite different from the language they use in their non-working lives. This process begins as soon as students start training and it is a powerful tool which helps health professionals feel connected to each other and part of the medical world. Unfortunately, the jargon, abbreviations and phrases that bind one group together shut other people out. We regularly meet professionals who argue that everyone knows what a contraction is or what 'ultrasound' means. That is not our experience. When was the last time the cervix was discussed at your dinner table?

Many medical terms have a familiar equivalent that will convey the meaning equally well: 'Pain relief' does not mean exactly the same as 'analgesia', or 'bleeding' the same as 'haemorrhage' but each is a more than adequate substitute. Other medical terms have lay equivalents: uterus/womb; placenta/afterbirth; amniotic fluid/the waters. However, replacement here is not so straightforward. You may want parents to learn medical terminology for a variety of reasons. For some parents, using the technical terms helps them feel more in control, just as it does for health professionals. When parents know technical words, it empowers them. Not only can they ask questions and understand the answers, they also elicit different behaviour in the health professionals they meet. 'How far has my cervix dilated?' prompts a different answer than 'Is it opening up?'.

If you want people to learn a medical term, you will need to offer them many repetitions. You need to say 'cervix, that ring of muscle like a drawstring at the neck of the uterus or womb'; or make a fist and hold it over your pubic bone every single time you use the word for the first week or so in a settled group (and every time you introduce the term in a changing group). It will help the group learn a new word if you offer several different explanations of it and say both the word and its informal definition in exactly the same tone of voice.

As well as finding ways of describing medical procedures and translating medical terms, antenatal teachers need to decide what language to use when talking about intimate human activities such as sex and excretion. We have been taught to be embarrassed about these subjects and they are often referred to rather indirectly, coyly, in a jokey way or not at all. Some health professionals respond by using rather formal terms and expressions which can sound stilted and may well not be understood. Others use euphemisms, and a few use more graphic terms commonly referred to as four letter words.

What words will you use to talk about sex? Will you use anatomical terms? Will you talk about making love? sexual intercourse? Having sex? Or will you use one of the many euphemisms that abound? What words will you use for male and female sex organs?

What words will you use when talking about excretion? Going to the toilet? The loo? Passing water? Urine? Having a pee? Doing a wee? Having a motion? Opening your bowels? It's vital to use words you are comfortable with, otherwise you will just convey embarrassment or tension.

As well as identifying words that you can use freely, you need to think about the people in your classes. What words will they understand and be able to relate to? Finding the right pitch takes practice and means observing the responses you get. It may also mean that you have to adapt your language and your attitudes!

If you find some words difficult, practice saying them out loud in private. Then say them out loud in front of a mirror. You may decide some words are not for you and that is fine. However, they may be right for others. It is important to be open-minded and flexible, so you can remain relaxed if someone in your class uses words that you would not use yourself.

Use analogies and metaphors

Use these figures of speech whenever you can and keep your eyes and ears open for any new ones parents offer you. You will soon have a collection of colourful phrases describing familiar experiences and feelings that parents *can* imagine to link them to more unfamiliar ones to come. Thus, having a caesarian under epidural anaesthesia can feel like 'someone doing the washing up in your tummy'; stitches can feel like 'sitting on a hedgehog'; carrying active twins can feel like 'a box full of puppies'; precipitate labour can feel like 'being in a tumbledrier'; a postnatal tummy rather resembles a 'half-set jelly'; and an unborn baby whose membranes are intact can be described as being 'in his or her own little space-craft'.

You may find some of these expressions distasteful or argue that what they describe is just as unfamiliar as the pregnancy experience they mirror. But they are colourful and stick in parents' minds, make people laugh and they get the point across. Such expressions are easier to use in a group where parents can be invited to give their reactions and feelings upon hearing them. Although they may evoke strong reactions, we find that in the long run, parents are more distressed when they are denied vivid, realistic descriptions than when they are offered them.

Perhaps the most fruitful use of metaphor comes when describing the inevitability and accelerating pattern of labour contractions. Here are some that parents have offered us over the years:

> . . . like standing beside a high speed railway track and you could hear the train far away then closer and closer then a tremendous whoosh of noise and speed as it passed then fading away again, leaving your heart pounding.
>
> . . . like one whole symphony squashed into a minute with the loud bits in the middle and lots of kettle drums.
>
> . . . like standing up to my knees in water and seeing the waves coming then crashing over me then fading out up on the beach and me not running away.
>
> . . . like a roller-coaster ride with the big bit getting higher all the time.
>
> . . . like letting go at the top of a helter-skelter . . . you just have to keep going till it ends.

The effect of individual words

Euphemisms have no place in helping parents prepare for birth. Saying 'discomfort' when you really mean 'pain', describing forceps only as 'the doctor's helping hands' or glossing over the mechanics of how a scalp electrode is attached leaves parents *less* prepared for these events than if you say nothing at all. All of us do this sometimes when our energy level is low or we don't have the support we need to offer hard truths to parents. But if you find yourself repeatedly shying away from telling things as they really are, you are probably doing so for your own needs not those of the parents.

You can be truthful without choosing the starkest words or the darkest slant on things. A scalp electrode may indeed be 'screwed into the baby's head', but a less emotive phrase like 'clipped on' will do just as well. Some words just sound more painful, like 'cut' (rather than 'snip') to describe an episiotomy or 'spines' (the anatomically correct term) rather than 'these bony bits here on the pelvis'. Some phrases are habitual but very misleading. Doctors may say to each other, 'when the baby's head hits the pelvic floor', but to a mother, a nightmare image may flash through her mind. The tricky bit is finding the middle way where truth and sensitivity meet. This is a balancing act that takes constant monitoring.

Developing accurate, realistic descriptions

In antenatal classes you will often find it necessary to describe objects, events and feelings that are either outside parents' experiences or inside the mother's body. Of course, visual aids like photos or actual objects will help, but you will still be called upon to conjure up words to paint a realistic picture of things that are mysterious or hidden. Most antenatal teachers take a long time to develop a repertoire of suitable descriptions and word-pictures. Here's a pattern that works for us:

- *What is it?* One sentence is almost always enough if you think hard about what you want to describe. Waffle confuses and irritates the listener and can convey the message that you don't really want the other person to understand what you are talking about. If you need help to develop concise, clear descriptions, using everyday language, try Heather Welford's book, *Illustrated Dictionary of Pregnancy and Birth* (see Further Reading, page 154). Keep pruning your words until only the essentials remain. For example: 'Forceps are made of metal and are curved a bit like salad servers so that they fit round the baby's head, cheeks and chin.'
- *What will the parents senses tell them?* Include as many of their five senses as you can. What will the mother see? Hear? Smell? Touch?

Feel? Taste? In a mixed group, offer the same to fathers. And don't forget the baby. What will he or she experience? The more vivid and accurate these points are, the more real your description will become. Again, keep it short, never using three words when one will do.

- *Stick with the parents' point of view.* For example, when discussing forceps, instead of telling parents about the different kinds of forceps and offering details about how they are applied (something of use only to those applying them), you might talk about the clang forceps produce when picked up, what the father will see happening, the various sensations mothers describe when forceps are inserted and traction is applied, or what effects forceps might have on the baby's experience of birth.
- *What will everyone involved be doing?* First, describe things from the parents' point of view then, if it would increase parents' understanding, describe briefly what one or two others in the room will be doing. For example: 'Forceps are always done by a doctor and he or she may have to pull quite hard to ease the baby out as the mother pushes.' Or: 'If you have a caesarian, a paediatrician will be there waiting to check the baby when he or she is born.'

You can follow this pattern (What is it?, then What will parents see/hear/touch?, then What will they be doing?) for almost everything you are called upon to describe. How would you use these pointers to describe a caesarian under epidural anaesthesia? A Ventouse extraction? An episiotomy?

The best way to discover whether you have conveyed accurate and useful information is to listen carefully to what parents say after their baby's birth. Ask them about their experience. Notice the language they use. Find out if anything happened that they felt unprepared for. Ask them for their suggestions about what you could say in future classes.

9

Leading discussion

Many people find it impossible to learn and change without regular discussions. If, week after week, they sit and listen, ask a few questions, then go home with their thoughts locked inside, they can often feel frustrated and sometimes even angry.

Through discussion, people can express what they think or feel, and acknowledge shared problems or beliefs. They may even discover the first steps towards finding their own solutions to common worries or difficulties.

Good discussions need groundwork so that the group is ready to handle them. They also need an effective trigger to start them off. Once in progress, the teacher needs to use subtle choreography to keep things going. The group members will be working hard too, preparing to speak, expressing themselves and listening to what others have to say.

Each new group you lead will have to learn these skills anew, but you can think ahead, anticipating certain fundamentals that apply to most discussions. Suggestions offered in this chapter will either remind you of things you already do or of things you would like to do. They will need to be adapted and changed to fit your own style and the needs of the particular group you are working with.

Thinking about discussion

While many antenatal teachers welcome discussion, some worry about losing control. It might never get started, it will take up too much time, it might get out of hand, or topics might be raised that would be hard to handle. How do you feel about discussion? What has your experience been?

Taking time to explore your own feelings and to improve your skills in starting and maintaining discussion can be very worth while. Discussions offer benefits that cannot be achieved through any other groupwork methods. And they are particularly suitable for adults, with their wide range of experiences, facts and beliefs to draw upon.

Laying the groundwork for discussion

Unless you get the preparation right, a discussion will not come to life. Good preparation includes:

- *Helping them interact as a group*. At a minimum, ensure that each person knows the name of several others and has spoken to several of the people present in small groups of three or four. In this way people discover ideas and attitudes of others in safety, before they are called upon to express their own in a larger group. Clarifying group rules and demonstrating by your approach that they are working are also important. Chapter 6 suggests ways to turn your class into a group.
- *Organizing appropriate sized groupings*. An ideal group size for many discussions is between six and 12 people. Fewer than six people have only a small range of experiences and ideas to draw on. They are more likely to get stuck or polarized between widely differing views. More than 12 people often have too much information and variety to keep track of easily. Participants may feel overwhelmed or confused.

  In a large group, the discussion process itself is also difficult unless each person is committed to listening to everyone else and each one takes only 1/14th or 1/16th of the amount of time and attention available. In practice, few groups are able or willing to do this; either a few people speak, taking all the time, or breakaway subgroups form. Pages 47–49 suggest ways of subdividing a large group.
- *Encouraging the habit of speech* Being an audience and listening for any length of time makes people lose the urge to speak. You can help break the silence barrier by getting people to talk in pairs or fours before starting a larger group discussion.

Starting a discussion

When you start a discussion you are *inviting* the group to join in. The warmer your invitation, the more likely they will be to respond. The group will judge your offer by both the words you say and the way in which you say them. Non-verbal messages include:

- *Posture.* Do you lean forward slightly, with a relaxed and open posture, and turn your body to face various people in the group including those to your immediate left and right?
- *Tone of voice.* When you ask a question, does your voice sound quizzical and genuinely interested in their response? Is the question asked slowly enough, with enough pauses between phrases to allow them to take it in and understand what you are asking?
- *Eye contact.* Do your eyes roam the group, making and breaking eye contact with many members, ready to catch the eye of someone willing to respond?
- *Silences.* Do you give them time to respond? If the gap between your question and the first word from them bothers you, try silently counting to 20 – slowly – while you continue to offer eye contact and an inviting expression. That may keep you busy while they gather themselves to speak.

Besides non-verbal cues, you will also use words to launch a discussion. Often, this means asking them a question. This needs careful thought as only some questions are effective discussion starters. Questions can be divided into several categories.

Closed questions

These questions usually have a right or a wrong answer or invite a 'yes' or a 'no' in response. The person asking the question often knows in advance what the answer is likely to be. Closed questions have very little place in antenatal classes and are no use for starting discussion. Some teachers may see such questions as encouraging and will probably offer them with all the inviting non-verbal cues described above.

'Who can tell me the three ways that labour starts?'
'What do you know about pain relief, then?'
'What's the best thing to do when a baby cries?'

These questions put parents on the spot and expose them to the possibility of admitting ignorance in public. Whatever parents say, they are bound to know less than the asker does and so feel silly. Some won't mind that, but many will mind a great deal. The wariest ones probably remember similar 'traps' from their schooldays. Often, these are the people you would most like to encourage to join in.

Leading questions

These can express the questioner's prejudices: 'Is anyone here really going to bottle feed?' or give a clear indication of the answer the asker wants: 'So what do you think about manufacturers making vast profits selling tiny sized baby clothes that are outgrown after the first two weeks?' Neither of these approaches is helpful.

Open questions

These are the most effective questions for triggering discussion. Your question will probably be 'open' only if

- it cannot be answered with 'yes' or 'no';
- it has more than one answer;
- you have no idea what the answer might be;
- it invites others to say as much or as little as they wish.

Open questions need planning and practice. Think first about the purpose of the discussion you are trying to start, then tailor your question to fit whatever aim you have in mind.

- *If you want them to explore their attitudes and feelings, try questions like:*

  'What are you most looking forward to in this pregnancy?'

  'What thoughts and images flashed through your mind when you first had a scan?'

  'Which bits about being in hospital will you find the hardest?'

  'How do you think your baby would want to be born?'

- *If you want them to talk about whatever is important for them in a particular topic, ask questions like:*

  'If I said, 'A woman's place is in the home', I'd probably get an argument! But where's a man's place in the early days after birth?'

'What have you heard about caesarian birth? Anything that made you uneasy?'

'If your baby advertised in the newspaper's Situations Vacant section for a mother or father, what do you think he/she would put in the ad?'

- *If you want them to discover shared experiences, ideas, or worries try asking:*

'Suppose you met someone who was trying to get pregnant and she asked, "What are the first three months like?" . . . what would you definitely mention?'

'Some women are sure they want drugs for pain relief and some are just as sure they don't. What about you?'

'Has anyone had any really vivid dreams? What's that like?'

- *If you want them to take the first steps towards finding their own answers, questions like these may start the process:*

'How do you think you might feel about breastfeeding when you are with other people?' (followed a bit later by) 'Are there people you would feel comfortable with?' (then) 'Are there any with whom you might feel uncomfortable?' (then finally) 'What could you do now to smooth the difficulties?'

'When you have had a similar problem in the past, what have you tried that might work here, too?'

'Three people have mentioned in-laws visiting in the first few days. How do you feel about this?'

Check that the questions you ask link with their own experiences. Asking first-time parents, 'How will you cope in the first few days?' will draw blank looks. But asking, 'What have you seen your friends doing that made you think "I definitely won't do that!"' may get them going.

Always try to link problems they may face in the future with those they have already faced in the past: 'What decisions have you already made for this baby? How are those choices the same and different from the choices you make for the baby during labour?'

Choosing which question to ask

To be effective, your questions should match the level of comfort and intimacy achieved by the group. Early in a group's life, early in a particular session, or even throughout the life of an open group (where members come and go week by week), some topics may be too hot to handle. If you bring them up, the group will either refuse to discuss them or be left feeling threatened and unhappy. (These topics are discussed in greater detail in Chapter 19.) A newish group may be willing to tackle cooler issues like the physical changes they noticed in early pregnancy, what they plan to buy for the baby, or all the ways they have heard of labours starting. In time, you can try more adventurous topics. Of course, what *you* think is a straightforward topic can and does bring all kinds of responses so be prepared to be surprised!

Judging the level of group comfort and intimacy takes practice. One of the best clues is to pay attention to your own feelings – are you starting to relax with them or is it still hard work to get them going? And pay attention to the group. Observe their body language – tense and anxious or settled and at ease? How are they dealing with silences – able to leave them for a bit or still rushing in to fill any you leave? Are they beginning to listen to each other with interest, turning to look when someone speaks and following the next person's response? Have they started to volunteer information, including their feelings and beliefs? And how have the rest reacted? Changes in their behaviour mirror changes in how they are feeling in the group.

Keeping discussion going

Many groups discuss well without a leader. You still need to keep an eye on the general atmosphere, assessing the level of energy in the room and watching for signs of anxiety or boredom. If there are several small groups working at the same time, would they benefit from a discreet visit to check that everyone feels safe and at ease? Listen for drops in noise level that might signal time to draw things to a close.

At other times you will take part in discussions as a member of the group, albeit one with the special role as the teacher. If the group seems unwilling to let you stop taking the lead, help them by reflecting back their questions:

'That's interesting . . . anyone have some thoughts on that?'
'I can see you would be curious about what I would do, but I'm not you.'

Acknowledge the requests for information and postpone them for later. Avoid correcting misinformation yourself. Instead, invite others to offer their thoughts or experiences and continue to ask open questions. If these techniques don't allow the group to turn to each other, you might leave them to get on without you. That often frees them to talk and listen.

You may need to intervene more actively if particular members of the group are preventing good discussion. If you can deal with such difficulties as a problem *for the group* and not yours alone, the better the outcome of any intervention. One way to do this is through group rules. Establishing early, for example, the idea that everyone deserves equal time will allow the more talkative to begin to monitor their contributions and will encourage others to take their share. If some do not, this can be aired with the whole group in neutral, non-judgemental ways. 'Remember a few weeks back when we set up the rules for this group (produce chart with them written down). How are we doing at keeping them?'

Another way is to reflect back to the group what you see happening and ask their help: 'When we are working in small groups everyone joins in, but in the big group only a few voices are heard. Shall we stick to small groups or can we do anything about the bigger ones?' Another approach is to be patient and wait for others to intervene, 'Oh Sally, not the story of your stitches again!'

If you do intervene, help the group to be aware of what you are doing. For example, someone may again and again tell stories of her last labour. One way to help her (and the group) move on is to overtly set aside time for her and anyone else to do this with the full attention of the group. The speaker must know how long she has and that she will not be interrupted. Often this is all that is needed, but should anyone continue to take more than the fair share of time, you can make time for her outside the group.

You may decide you need to be more direct in your intervention either because time is short or the person has not responded to other attempts. When you do, choose a way that neither puts that person down nor involves you in an argument with them. Unless you do, you will lose the trust of the group even if you 'win' that particular encounter. Below are things you might do or say to intervene if individuals are persistently unhelpful in group discussions.

The ones who speak often and at great length

- Suggest the group follows the rule where no one speaks twice before everyone has spoken once.
- Sit next to those you wish to quieten, so they find it harder to catch your eye.
- Intervene. Say, 'Thank you Alan. Now let's see if others have a view on this.'
- Break them into smaller groups so everyone has time to talk.
- Say, 'Well I know what Kathleen, Mary and Sue think about this but I don't know how it is for the rest of you. What was going through your minds in the last few minutes?'

The ones who never speak

- Catch their eye and invite them in, 'Anyone else have a view on this?' (Don't address anyone by name – it's too threatening.)
- Quickly ask the same question of several people. Include the silent person if you feel she would *like* to speak as she will probably be rehearsing an answer when the others respond.
- Set up a round where everyone speaks.
- Break into smaller groups so the silent ones feel more able to speak.
- Use a safe pot or trigger pictures (see Chapter 10).
- Respect the fact that some people do not wish to contribute and that this does not necessarily mean they are not benefiting from being in the class.

Clowns and jokers

- Accept the off-the-cuff quip then ask again. 'Well yes, it might be like popping a cork out of a bottle but what if it's not like that?'
- Ask questions that acknowledge the *real* feelings and fears behind the jokes. Sometimes, ask the close-to-the-bone questions of the jokers first. 'How do you think you might really feel if that happened?'

- Ask them to hold back. 'Can we come back to that later and start by covering the things that are more likely to happen?'

The ones who never listen

- Don't allow interruptions. 'Hang on, Theresa. Can you just wait until Gill's finished?'
- Suggest she takes the role of charting what the group is doing.
- Remind the group of the rules about listening with respect.

Try not to get into the position where you are coping with people's unhelpful behaviour while the group sits back and watches with interest while you struggle. If you find it a problem, they do too, so they have just as much interest in getting it right as you do.

Managing strong feelings

Sometimes a discussion allows parents to acknowledge or express deep feelings and worries. People may cry, become angry or express great joy during the course of a discussion, and in this way they allow others to see how things really are for them. The important thing to remember is that discussions do not *cause* these feelings, they may just provide a rare opportunity for them to be expressed.

Strong feelings and negative thoughts are worth airing because they tend to fester when left unspoken or buried at the back of people's minds. By allowing people to express their feelings and maybe to cry, you are offering them a chance to let off steam, release anxiety and begin to hold the issue up to the light so they can look at it with some perspective.

There are several things you can do to help individual members (and the group as a whole) to feel safe and supported both during the expression of powerful feelings and afterwards as the group moves on:

- Acknowledge what is happening calmly and sympathetically. 'This is a painful memory for you.'
- If it is appropriate, move closer to the person who is expressing strong feelings, to support them rather than to stop them (Figure 9.1).
- Remember tears can be infectious and that if one person starts to cry, others might well join in.

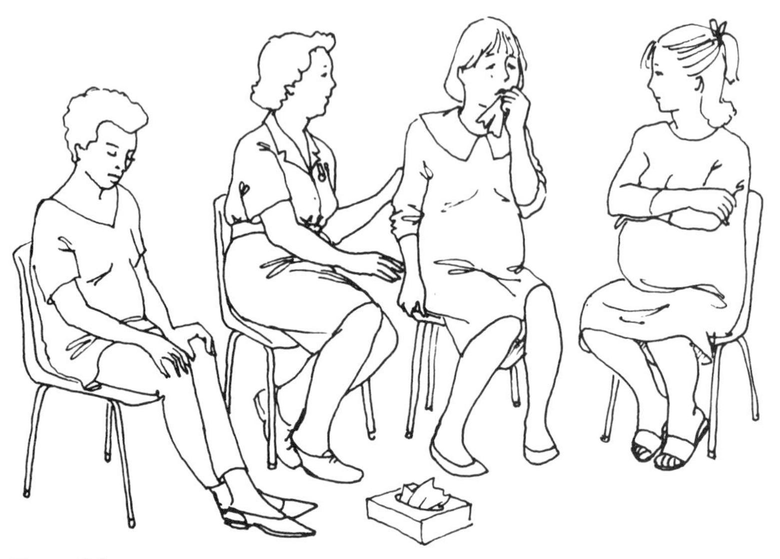

Figure 9.1

- Avoid the temptation to reassure. If their fears are totally unfounded you can put them into perspective later.
- Allow time, balancing the needs of the individual with those of the group.
- If necessary, offer the individual time after the class to talk further.
- Afterwards, acknowledge what has happened. If it has been hard for an individual or a group, it helps to say so briefly and with empathy. Then choose your next activity with care so that the atmosphere is gently lightened.

Bringing discussion to an end

When a discussion is drawing to a close, you may find you need to help the group sum up what has happened and to lift the group mood if the discussion touched on matters that were painful or controversial. Both are important for finishing a discussion well.

Summing up can be done by the teacher or by group members. If you sum up, you need to pick out the salient points that have arisen and state them clearly and succinctly. If a group has touched on a painful or emotional topic, the mood is likely to be sombre and people may have mentally pulled away from the group. You need to acknowledge that it has been hard and then lift the gloom and bring them back together. One way to do this is to suggest they turn to the person next to them and say how the discussion was for them or the one word that is foremost in their mind. Then bring the whole group together to do something light and lively such as discussing what to take into hospital. Or put on the kettle and take a short social break.

Initiating and maintaining discussion is like an adventure. You cannot predict what will happen. Like adventures, discussions can carry risk, but the benefits of giving people time to share their feelings and develop their thoughts and ideas are well worth the effort.

10

Encouraging active learning

People learn best by taking an active part in the learning process. When they have opportunities to discover information and ideas for themselves, people remember better and are more likely to be able to put their new knowledge into use (see Chapter 3).

So, taking time to develop activities that encourage people to participate and think for themselves will enhance the effectiveness of your classes.

Thinking ahead

Identifying your aims

Before you decide to include active learning techniques in your class, or if you are already using them, take some time to think through what you are aiming to achieve.

- Are you reinforcing information that you have already covered?
- Are you using the activity to change the pace and atmosphere in the class?
- Do you intend to stimulate discussion?
- Are you hoping to raise awareness of new issues?

You may have very different purposes at different points in the course and you will need to tailor the activity so that it achieves your aim.

Laying the foundations

A class that has been an audience will be far less likely to respond positively to an invitation to participate than a class that has already become a group. People need to know each other, be used to contributing their thoughts and ideas and, above all, be confident that any contribution they make will be accepted and welcomed. So if you want active participation, you need to set the scene right from the beginning of the course (see Chapter 6).

The size of your class

Nearly all activities work best in small groups, so if you have a large class you will need to plan how you will divide people up (pages 47–49 offer several ways). As you will not be able to be present at every small group all the time, you will need to decide which activities are suitable for groups to work on without your guidance. Then work out ways of giving them the necessary instructions and ways of ensuring that all goes well – that instructions are understood and followed and that queries and questions get answered. You might write out brief instructions on cards, or print them on a flipchart. While people are working together, you could join each group briefly and if necessary answer questions or make suggestions.

Where in the course?

It is important that the activity you introduce links with the topics you are covering and the information you are giving. When you are planning where to place an activity, ask yourself:

- Does it enhance and build on what you have already done?
- Does it give a wider picture or encourage people to look further forward?

The optimum time for many activities is after a topic has been discussed or explained. The activity then offers people a chance to explore or handle the information in a different way. They can assess their understanding, learn from each other and have the experience of putting their ideas and information into practice.

Ensuring relevance

Your activities will be effective only if they are relevant to the people in your classes. Suppose you devised an activity around going back to work – this would fall flat with a group of under-18s. If you have people from ethnic minorities in your classes, do your activities reflect their culture and way of life? If you teach teenagers, single or adoptive parents, do the activities you use address the issues they are facing? If you teach couples, is the father's perspective included?

Introducing active learning

The way you introduce activities is important. Although they can be likened to games, it may be unwise to introduce them as such because the word has mixed connotations. For some, the idea of 'playing games' sounds childish; others may feel manipulated. You will need to think of ways of inviting people to try something new that will stimulate interest and sound inviting. Your tone of voice and body language are probably as important as the words you use.

Developing activities

There are an infinite number of activities you can devise and adapt. It can be great fun and very rewarding to invent your own. Keep them simple and think about the appearance of the 'props' you use. For example, if you use written cards make sure the writing is clear and legible. Pictures should be up-to-date and kept clean and neat. You may find it useful to mount statements and pictures on stiff card, then cover them with transparent plastic.

Practice

Before using an activity in class, try it out with a group of friends or colleagues and ask them to give you feedback. Did it achieve your aim? Did they enjoy it? What did they learn? Were your instructions clear? What improvements could be made?

Feedback

When you have tried an activity in class, take time to notice the reactions of the participants. You could also ask them what they got out of it. Then review and, if necessary, adapt what you are doing so that it becomes more effective.

The rest of the chapter outlines some activities that we have used regularly with antenatal groups. You can adapt them or build on them. We hope they will prompt your own inventions.

Activities to check and reinforce information

Ordering activities

There are many procedures and features of birth that follow or are likely to follow a more-or-less predictable order. You can help people reinforce their understanding and share their information by writing out the possible components of a procedure or event, one item on each card. Then invite small groups to work together to place them in a line that mirrors the order in which they are likely to happen. One or two cards might be rejected straight away and you can follow on by clarifying why this was done and by discussing any other issues that arise. For example:

- The following boxed items all *could* happen to a woman being induced. Can the group sort them into a likely order?

> A drip with oxytocin – acupuncture – a pessary – a sweep – making love – walking about – breaking the waters – castor oil – nipple stimulation – raspberry leaf tea.

- Can the group sort the cards in the next box into the events they think might happen should they opt for a physiological third stage, and those they would expect in a managed one?

> pulling on the cord – clamping the cord – upright posture – midwife's hand over the pubic bone – no waiting for the next contraction – baby to the breast – allowing the cord to stop pulsing – injection of syntometrine – no touching the uterus.

Recognition activities

You can help people check their information and identify differences by displaying a series of photographs or charts. Then lead a discussion in a way which ensures nobody is put on the spot or feels he or she has got it wrong.

- Can they match a photograph of a health professional in uniform (midwife, house-officer, care assistant, health visitor, etc.) to the appropriate title on another card?
- Can they sort a pile of photographs of breastfeeding babies into those that are well latched on and those that are not?
- Can they spot the differences in charts showing 36 and 40 weeks gestation?

Solving problems

Short 'case histories', which describe real people facing dilemmas, offer people an opportunity to apply the information you have just given them.

Jane says: 'Simon, wake up. It's four o'clock and I just woke up and the bed is all wet. What should we do?'

Ian says: 'She's going to have that pethidine after all. Now what was it I was meant to do to help?'

Mark says: 'She's been hard at it for hours now and I'm exhausted. How can I help myself get through the night?'

Sophie says: 'I have to decide whether to have an epidural or a general for a caesarian birth and I can't remember anything they said about it in classes. What are the advantages for each?'

Drawing your own conclusions

These activities offer people opportunities not only to check their knowledge, but also to practise making decisions in situations where a variety of things may happen. They can also demonstrate the importance of being flexible and being able to adapt to the different patterns that labour and birth can take.

To show parents how changing and subjective such decisions are, you could put various pieces of information on cards, turn all of them face down and invite one person to turn them over one by one, 'telling the story' according to each new bit of information (Figure 10.1).

In the case of the onset of labour, a variety of things could happen in a variety of sequences. You could have one card for each of the items in the box opposite. Then invite one member of a group of four to lay the cards out, face down, in a vertical line. In whatever order they come, the cards 'tell a story' - somebody's labour probably started like

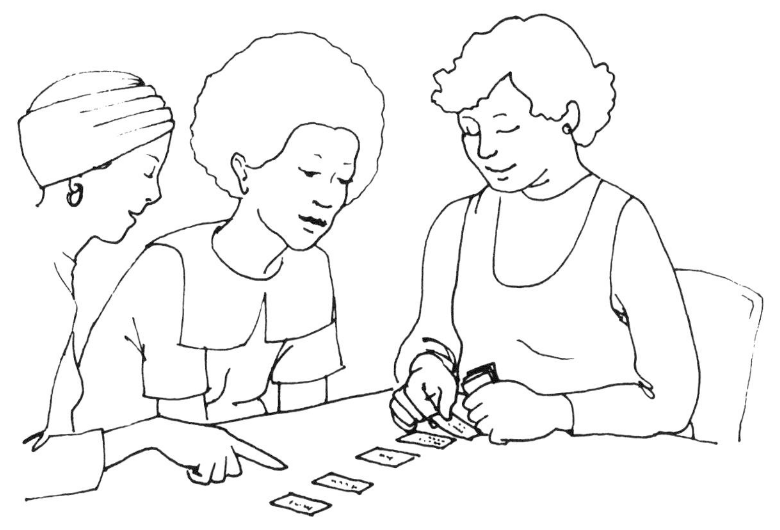

Figure 10.1

that! Start at the top of the cards, and turn over a card and start the story. Ask her to keep turning up cards and stop the moment she feels 'Yes, I am in labour' or 'No, oh dear, false alarm. I'll have to wait for another day'. When she has decided, she collects the cards, shuffles them and lays them out for the next person to 'tell the story' and decide 'Am I in labour?'

> Ouch! with a contraction – a contraction every 10 minutes – four contractions in the last hour – no change in contractions – definite gush of water down the woman's leg – a show – wet knickers – contractions lasting 10 seconds – contractions lasting 30 seconds – contractions lasting 45 seconds – contractions getting stronger – diarrhoea – can still chat and watch tv during contractions – seven minutes since the last contraction.

You could also use a 'Labour Line'. Write on separate cards a variety of things that could happen from the start of labour to the end. These should include

- Obstetric events such as the use of electronic fetal monitors, pethidine or Entonox.

- Physiological events experienced by the mother like vomiting, pressure on the rectum or the shakes. Include cards for contractions of varying lengths from 10 seconds to a full minute or more.
- Feelings, both positive and negative, that parents can experience during labour. For example, boredom, anxiety, exhaustion, excitement, tears of joy and so on. If you are unsure about what to include, think back to the feelings you have experienced when looking after a woman who had a long labour – and add them!
- Events – including, of course, the birth of the baby, but also everyday things like a cup of tea and phone calls to in-laws. You can even put in cards that say things like 'oh dear' or 'I've had enough'.
- You may need to repeat some items such as 'contractions getting stronger' on several cards.

Then organize the class into small groups of four or five and pass each group a complete pack. Ask each person to take a handful of cards and lay them out in a single line in the order that reflects their view of what might happen in labour. Initially, each person works independently, adding cards to the group line in whatever order she or he thinks appropriate.

When all cards are placed in a line, ask the group to stand back and look. Do they want to move anything? Invite them to talk about which cards could go elsewhere. This promotes discussion and enables people to check the information they have acquired during the course. If several groups are working at the same time, the end results are bound to be different. This can be a graphic demonstration of the unpredictable pattern of labour and the advantages of being able to respond flexibly.

These and similar activities allow the group opportunities to review what they have been told and to discuss ideas among themselves. If they can do them, it will be clear proof to them (and to you) that they have learned. Activities also give members of the group who are less quick to pick up knowledge a second chance in a safe, supportive way.

Raising awareness – initiating discussion

There are several activities that can be used to start discussion as well as the open questions reviewed in Chapter 9. These include:

- *Drawings*. No matter what their skill in drawing, many people find this a useful way to clarify what they are thinking and feeling now and how they might feel in the future. In order for people to feel confident and safe enough to try this rather unusual way of working in the group, it is very important to stress that artistic talent is not important, and that what they draw will not be commented on by anyone else.

Provide each person with paper and pencil and invite them to do a drawing (or series of drawings) that represents, for example, how they are feeling about the pregnancy, how they imagine labour might be, or what life will be like with a new baby. If they want to, each person can describe their own picture to the group. It is up to you to ensure that your introductory promise is fulfilled and that nobody analyses or comments on anyone else's picture or on what the drawer chooses to say about it.

- *The 'safe pot'*. Because people are often reluctant to talk about the things that really concern or frighten them, it is helpful to offer them a way to raise these issues anonymously.

  Provide a container – the 'safe pot' – and paper and pencils. Invite people to write down the topics they would like covered in the course, including the things that most worry them . Stress that there is no need to give their names or say which their topic is. Ask them to place their papers in the safe pot. You can then draw out the papers one at a time and lead a discussion on the chosen topic. Alternatively, you can ask people in turn to draw out and read aloud a topic. Then open out the discussion to include everyone. If you have a number of topics to cover you may want to do some in each class, ensuring that by the end of the course, all of them have been included.

Is there life after birth?

One of the challenges the antenatal teacher faces is helping parents to see beyond labour and birth to parenthood. Part I of the book covers this issue generally; here, we suggest various ways of helping parents see over the 'wall' of birth to focus on life with a baby. Many of these examples can be adapted to apply to the antenatal period and for labour as well.

Trigger pictures

This activity can be used to promote discussion on information you have already covered or to raise new issues. First, choose one particular aspect of birth or parenting (e.g. labour or life in hospital). Make a list of the various issues that people would find useful to think about in advance. For example, in the postnatal period, these might include: breast changes, breastfeeding, a crying baby, weighing the baby, being in the postnatal ward, coming home for the first time, coping with extra washing, being woken in the night, and so on.

Then, collect photos or pictures from magazines and newspapers which are likely to trigger thinking and promote discussion on these points. When choosing pictures, look for bright, clear drawings or photographs. Adverts can be surprisingly useful if you cut out the text. Make sure the pictures you choose reflect the cultures, ethnic groups and lifestyles that are relevant to the people in your class and ensure that the father's perspective is specifically included. You may need to search a little for pictures that portray parents and babies from some ethnic groups other than your own. One way of approaching this is to enlist the help of your class, asking them for photos or old magazines and newspapers that are published specifically for that section of the community.

Don't limit your imagination. We ourselves have included some unlikely pictures. One, of a slice of rich, inviting gateau, evokes a range of responses from 'Birth is a celebration ' to 'How will I ever get my figure back?' A picture of a packet of sanitary towels can raise discussion on lochia, what it is, how long it lasts and so on. A picture of a condom, dutch cap or pack of contraceptive pills leads you neatly into contraception and sex after birth.

Having prepared your set of pictures and decided when in the course to use them, lay them face down on the floor and invite individuals to turn one over and say what it makes her or him think of. It is very important to accept every reaction you get, even if it is quite unexpected. Then open out the discussion to include everyone. Then it is someone else's go to turn over a picture.

Lucky dip

This is a variation of 'trigger pictures' and achieves much the same aim. Collect a variety of items that are relevant to life after birth – eight to 12 items will be ample. These might include: a breast pad, a nappy (disposable, terry or both), a dummy, a feeding bottle, or a room thermometer. How about a pair of lacy knickers which might start discussion about getting your figure back or sex after birth? Or a novel or magazine to make them to wonder if there will ever be time to put their feet up and read? A clock might prompt a range of questions about feeding schedules, having time to get everything done or waking in the night.

Having collected your chosen items, place them in a large container like a nappy bucket and invite people, one at a time, to pick out an item and say whatever comes to mind. Then broaden out the discussion.

The 24-hour clock

This device helps parents to focus on the dramatic changes a baby makes to day-to-day routine. It works best if it is done after a discussion on breastfeeding so that parents are already aware of the frequency of feeds.

Provide each person (fathers as well) with a sheet of paper on which are drawn two 24-hour clocks (Figure 10.2). Ask everyone to fill in

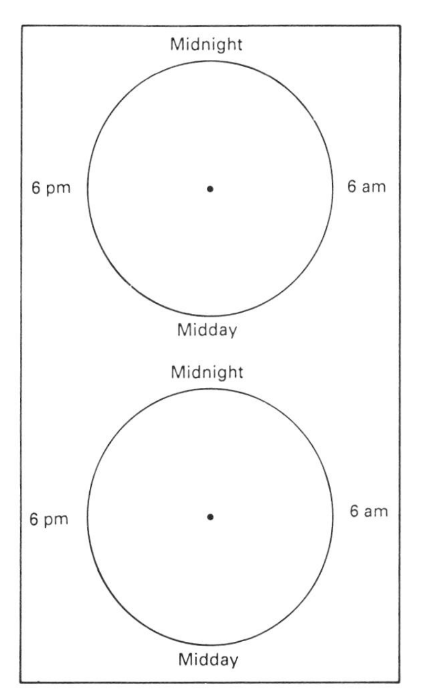

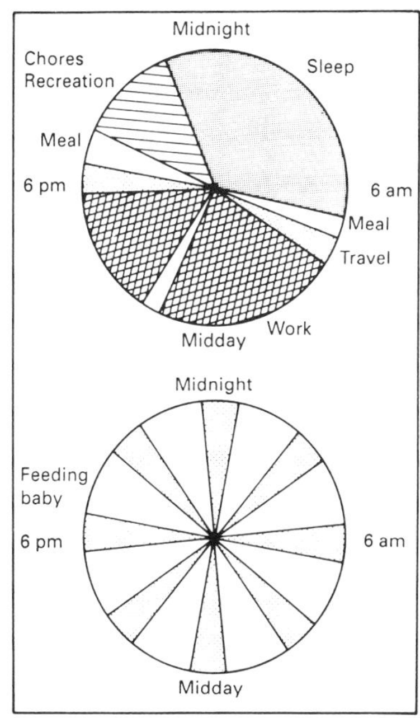

Figure 10.2

wedges of time that correspond to the way they spend their time at the moment. They may want to choose one day in the last week and allocate each task or activity a wedge of time. Suggest they include cooking and other household chores, work, travel, socializing and relaxing as well as sleep. It often helps if you demonstrate by filling in your own chart.

Then ask everyone to imagine that their baby is three weeks old. What will life be like then? Remind them about the number of feeds a baby is likely to need in 24 hours and the length of time they might spend with the baby from the time they pick her up to the time she settles back to sleep. Suggest they put these wedges in first. Again you could demonstrate on your chart. Add any other babycare activities you may have discussed. When might they bath this baby? Then, if they haven't already done so, ask them to compare the two charts. Are there any differences? How will they fit everything in?

Many people feel overwhelmed when confronted with this scenario, so it is very important to follow up with opportunities to think out how they might manage their lives with these new and unpredictable demands on their time and energy. One way you can follow on is to use the next activity.

Priority sheets

Provide each person with a sheet, listing a range of common household and recreational activities. These could include jam making as well as essential cooking, washing curtains as well as clothes washing. Make sure that you include a range of recreational activities so that you can follow on with discussion about meeting the parents' needs for human contact, exercise and relaxation. Draw columns beside the list, labelled 'Essential', 'Important', 'Unimportant'.

Ask everyone to tick the items that they consider to be essential, those they consider important and those that are unimportant. Acknowledge that people will have different priorities. For some, it may be having the evening meal ready on time; for others, making sure the lavatory is clean even if the rest of the place is a tip could be 'essential'. Encourage couples to talk about their priorities with each other. They may discover they are very different. If these can be raised and talked through beforehand, so that some compromises might be reached, some of the frustrations and stresses of the first few weeks of parenthood can be reduced.

Finally, suggest they refer back to the 24-hour clock and think of ways of fitting the 'essentials' into the second pattern.

Buttons

This activity helps to demonstrate the subtle but profound relationship changes the arrival of a new baby brings. It is important to stress to the group that this is just a way of representing internal impressions so that they can be clarified and looked at. People also need to know that each time someone tries this activity, it will turn out differently because the way we feel about our relationships changes. It is also important to ensure that nobody comments on or tries to interpret anyone else's pattern.

Provide a large quantity of buttons of different shapes, sizes and colours. Then invite each person to make their own pattern by choosing buttons to represent themselves and other significant people in their lives. Ask them to place buttons on the floor in front of them in a pattern that best represents how they feel each individual relates to themselves and to each other *at this moment*. Encourage them to include emotionally significant friends and relatives even if they live at a distance or even abroad. Pets, too, can be included – especially dogs and cats.

When everyone has arranged their buttons to their satisfaction, you could suggest each person tells a partner who the buttons represent and why they are placed where they are. Then give give each person a small button to represent their baby to be placed within the pattern. 'Where does the baby fit into the picture? Do you need to make any changes in order to accommodate her or him? Does anyone move out? Does anyone move in?' Each person could then tell their partner about any buttons they moved when the 'baby' arrived.

You might consider using pink or blue buttons, but this might precipitate more than you bargained for if there are people in the class for whom the sex of their baby is a big personal or family issue.

There is no deep significance to be read into this activity. However, it does offer people an opportunity to focus on how they feel that the arrival of a new person might change things. Buttons can offer enormous variety of size, colour, shape and texture and it is fascinating to watch the absorption and care with which people select their buttons.

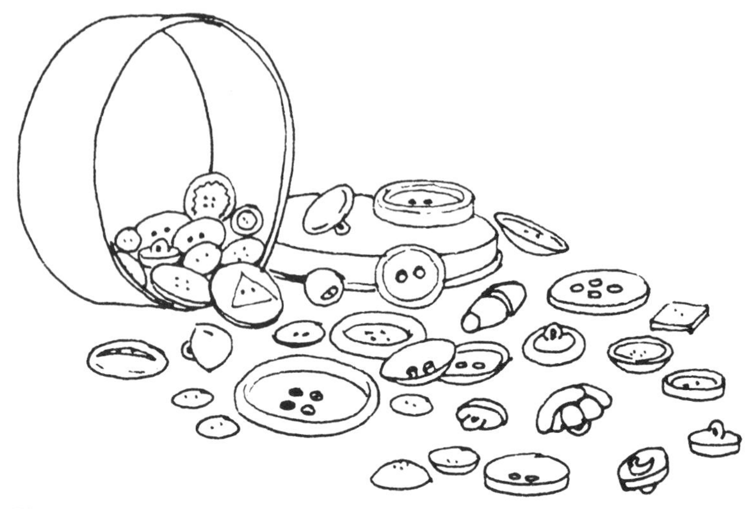

Figure 10.3

In conclusion

There are a large number of activities that could be used in classes. They are cheap and easy to produce and they add variety and spice to the course.

If they are well thought through and tailored to the participants' needs and cultures, they go beyond helping people to understand facts. They offer people a whole variety of opportunities to use new information; to solve problems; to identify issues that might become relevant to them; or to reach their own decisions. They can help prospective parents to realize how important it is to be flexible and open-minded about labour and parenting. They are one of the best ways to increase the group's confidence in their own strengths and abilities.

11

Teaching physical skills

Pregnancy, labour and new parenthood force women (and to some extent men) to use their bodies in new ways. This chapter is about helping them learn new skills to cope with the very physical side of giving birth and looking after a baby. We have called these 'physical skills' and there are dozens you might include in your classes. For example:

- ways to walk and stand;
- positions for comfort in labour;
- massage;
- various kinds of relaxation;
- breathing patterns;
- pelvic floor exercises;
- practical babycare skills from how to swaddle a newborn to how to mix a bottle;
- how to position and latch on a breastfed baby.

In addition, there are all the other possibilities you will find listed in Chapter 5. In fact, the issue that is likely to face you is not, 'What will I teach?' but 'What will I leave out until parents mention it?'

You have probably come across these skills or taught them yourself. If not, many of the books listed at the end of this section offer suggestions or you could hire videos or tapes from a Health Education Unit. Alternatively, you could arrange a PROSPECT workshop, which can be designed to meet the specific needs of staff in your area. Other people who could help include obstetric physiotherapists who are trained to teach a variety of physical skills, Active Birth teachers, National Childbirth Trust teachers, practitioners of the Alexander Technique and many independent midwives (see Useful Addresses in Appendix I). In the next three chapters, we focus on the skills that professionals most often ask us to work on with them.

Moving from information to mastery

Information – knowing what to do – is important, but it is not enough. If parents are going to feel confident enough to actually use the skills you teach, they need to feel that the skills actually belong to them. This can only happen if they try them out several times.

For instance, you might decide to teach positions for labour. One approach would be to describe six or seven positions, assume them yourself, guide a group member into various positions while the others watch, or pass out a handout illustrating them. In all these ways, you would give people the *information* that various positions are possible, but you give little else. If women have never tried these positions in advance, the chances that they will use them in labour when under stress, in an unfamiliar place and surrounded by strangers is virtually zero. Even after one practice, use rates will be very low.

However, if you decide that positions for labour are very important, you could include several practices in different classes, with a variety of explanations as to why they are useful. You might even give 'homework' although people almost never practise between sessions even if you urge them to do so and enquire how they got on. With frequent opportunities to practise over time, parents get the 'feel' of that skill and make it their own.

Parents will only have the time to practise and repeat a small number of skills during your course. By prioritizing, then checking postnatally, you can discover whether or not you chose the appropriate skills. Did parents actually use what you taught? Which were particularly helpful? What skills do they wish they had covered? Their answers will help you fine-tune your selections.

Setting the scene

Where you teach will have a direct impact on what physical skills you teach. Your job will be easier if everyone has a solid, movable chair without arms. Group members could bring a small pillow or two to make chairs more comfortable and adapt them to various uses (see Figure 12.1, page 127). A reasonably clean floor and a carpet are welcome extras because they encourage kneeling when experimenting with positions, relaxation or massage. If you can assure privacy and freedom from interruption, people will feel more willing to try some of the more out-of-the-ordinary things we teach in antenatal groups.

If your room falls short of these minimal requirements, modify it if you can. Movable screens can be used to improve privacy if the room is overlooked. Ask – persistently if necessary – for different chairs. If you are short of equipment, try approaching local voluntary groups for help. Where clean carpeting isn't available, most carpet merchants will offer offcuts and sample squares for little or nothing, giving each person his or her own soft patch of floor.

Don't worry if your teaching room is small or you don't have mattresses or a large supply of pillows. All the necessary physical skills, including relaxation, can be taught very effectively without these. The next chapter suggests ways of doing this.

Helping parents feel comfortable in their learning

Most of the physical skills you teach in antenatal classes are outside people's everyday experience. *You* may have suggested dozens of times that women sit on their hands and tighten the muscles in their vaginas to check if their buttocks tighten too. For you, such a suggestion is a commonplace, but for each new group it is unusual to say the least! Many of the skills you teach will involve parts of the body that are rarely if ever discussed in public. You may ask couples to touch each other in front of others or suggest to reluctant, tired pregnant women that they move to another position. In these and many other instances, you teach against resistance. Because of this, you need to accommodate modesty and cajole reluctant adults to do something they would rather not do. Here are some suggestions to make this admittedly difficult task easier:

Getting people started

Gentle but persistent encouragement will usually get even the most reluctant women into action and, once started, most are willing to continue. Acknowledge and sympathize with their lethargy.

Make all your instructions optional

Invite people rather than telling them: 'You might like to', or 'If your arms are crossed, you could try resting each hand on your knees'.

Start with skills that are probably safe

If you move from everyday things to the more intimate, people will begin to trust you and each other. For example, when teaching positions, start with pairs standing up. This loosens them up and allows most to go on to kneeling or squatting without too much unease. For massage, backs, shoulders and hands are relatively safe, while face-to-face work is more intimate. If you ask too much too quickly, people will baulk or feel too anxious to be able to learn. However, once they have tried safer things, do take some risks or you won't push them to learn new things to cope with the new challenges ahead.

Make sure you believe in the usefulness of everything you teach

Your conviction will come across to the group and increase their willingness to follow instructions.

Coping with non-participants

No matter how you approach trying out new physical skills, some people may never join in. They are free to opt out and will have all kinds of explanations for their reluctance. Some could hold cultural taboos against touching other people or against men and women touching in public. Perhaps the situation reminds them too strongly of past ridicule in PE lessons. Maybe they can't imagine sitting in a group with their knees wide apart or they are so frightened by the thought of giving birth that even *pretending* to do so is beyond their courage.

The only way to find out for sure what stops someone having a go, is to ask her or him. An open question (see Chapter 9) might help you understand or it may feel too much like prying. Only you can judge. If you decide to ask someone what is difficult for them, make sure you do it discreetly, so that they are not further embarrassed by being put on the spot in public. If you have been respectful and only asked them to do what you believe in, you have done all you can. By continuing to treat reluctant people with respect and including them whenever possible, you will find that some – though not all – will change their minds.

Making the most of everything you teach

When parents are practising physical skills in your class, they are doing several things besides learning the skill itself. They are helping the group become more lively and cohesive because sharing the experience of doing things always changes how people feel about each other. At the same time, you can give them a glimpse of the pressures and feelings to come. Perhaps they are trying to relax in a room full of strangers while ignoring the workmen outside the door – tell them that labour wards can be like that, too. Learning to feel centred, relaxed and at peace despite the surroundings will help them cope better with labour. Other analogies abound. Women may feel tired and unsure if they have the energy to try out second stage positions. However, caring for a new baby will mean doing things when they don't really want to. Discovering they can do so in your class may help them later when their baby's demands cannot be postponed. In the same way, asking couples to touch each other in public foreshadows the experience in the labour room. Reflecting on present experience and extrapolating to the future offers them much more than the basics of massage or breathing awareness.

For maximum effectiveness in teaching physical skills, here are some key points:

- Do them often, in short bursts of five or 10 minutes.
- Do them as and when they fit into the rest of the programme; avoid having to move rooms or change the teacher (see Chapter 15).
- Do them whenever you feel the group would benefit from a change of pace or injection of energy.
- Do them whenever the talk gets so gloomy that the group needs something practical and positive to get their teeth into.
- Do them often enough and in a variety of contexts so parents move from copying what they see to mastering the skill for themselves. If you do, you give parents a resource for the rest of their lives.

12

Relaxation

Most teachers consider that helping parents learn to relax is an essential part of the antenatal course. This chapter suggests ways in which you can integrate relaxation into every class and help parents practise it in many different ways.

Preparing to lead

The first step in effective teaching of relaxation starts long before the group meets – it starts with reviewing your own views on relaxation and the way you do or don't use it in your life. Whatever your outward approach, however carefully you structure your teaching and choose your words, your attitude to relaxation is likely to seep into everything you teach. We find that over the years, relaxation has taken a more important place in our lives and that has helped both of us feel more confident in what we teach parents.

Would you benefit from using the skills you teach in your everyday life at work and at home? How could you begin to use it regularly for yourself? What do you need to learn? What support and help might you need? Where and from whom could you get this?

Your feelings about relaxation in labour are also important. Have you been disillusioned by seeing women in labour who have been disappointed when relaxation has failed to bring them as much relief as they had hoped for? Or do you think relaxation is the key to meeting the challenge of labour?

Talking through your experiences and attitudes with someone else might help you clarify and understand your feelings.

When you begin to look for specific teaching skills, or review what you already do, there are plenty of books, tapes and courses with scripts and suggestions, many of them mentioned in the Further

Reading section at the end of Part II. In this chapter, we summarize a few approaches. We don't describe different relaxation techniques in depth, partly because there are other sources of this information but mainly because in order to be really familiar and at ease with a technique, you need first to have experienced it for yourself. So take every opportunity you can to participate in other people's relaxation sessions. Not only will you learn new techniques, you will enjoy the benefits for yourself. In addition, listen to tapes and read about other people's ideas. Then, because it never rings true when a teacher uses someone else's approach word-for-word, develop your own unique style, words and images.

You may find it helpful to practise with friends, family or colleagues. Lead them through a relaxation sequence then ask them to tell you what they liked about what you did and what they could suggest you improve. Or you can use a tape recorder. Afterwards listen to the tape as though it was someone else talking and identify what is good about it and what needs improving. Then try it again.

Making a place for relaxation

When planning your course, it is important to think about the timing of relaxation sessions within each class and within the course. Will you do some relaxation at every class? If not, how many times will you include it in the course? In order to acquire and develop this skill, people need practice. It is tempting to hope that, between each class, everyone goes home and practises assiduously. In reality, this will only happen if you are enthusiastic about relaxation and if you create opportunities in class for people to actually experience the pleasures and benefits for themselves. By having frequent and sometimes short sessions, and by using a variety of approaches, you offer them time for practice and an enjoyable experience which will help to maintain interest and awareness.

Where in the class will you put relaxation? Always in the same time slot, such as the beginning or end? Or will you use it flexibly, noticing what is happening in the group and putting it in where it seems appropriate?

How will you link relaxation to other topics in that class? This may be very difficult if relaxation is taught as a separate topic or even by a health professional other than the one who leads the rest of the course.

This way of working can reduce the impact of what we see as the central message about relaxation: that it is a core skill and can be part of everything. The ability to teach relaxation effectively can be learned by anyone who takes time and trouble to think through the issues, to make relaxation a part of her own life, to gather ideas and information, and to practise and develop this skill.

Introducing relaxation to the group

Just as you need to be personally aware of the usefulness of relaxation by using it in your own life, you also need to convince parents of the personal relevance in learning to relax. Acting on the assumption that relaxation is 'a good thing for pregnant women to learn, so let's just get on with it' may mean that many class members opt out of making this skill their own. A better method is to tailor your approach so that people actually enjoy the experience of learning to relax in class and to relate it in as many ways as possible to people's real lives, both now and as they will be in the future. Here are a few examples of the benefits of relaxation. It:

- brings peace and a sense of well being;
- improves posture;
- reduces stress;
- increases effectiveness at home and at work;
- conserves energy;
- helps with insomnia;
- makes for safer drivers;
- aids successful breastfeeding;
- helps to reassure distressed babies;
- *and it feels wonderful!*

Relaxation can also be the central peg from which the skills and attitudes specific to labour can be rooted (see box opposite).

Another good way of establishing relevance is to invite people who use relaxation to talk about how it fits into their lives and the benefits they feel. Those with no experience could be asked to talk about the situations that make them tense and 'achy' and which they would like to change. Encourage people to identify where their particular tension

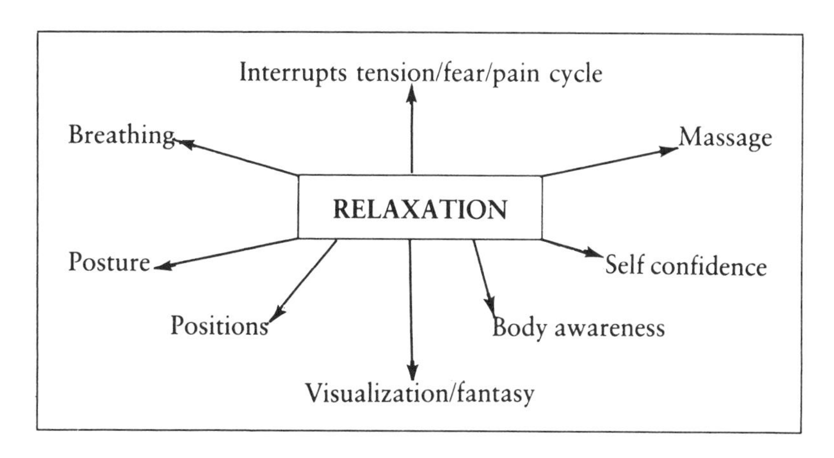

points are and suggest they could spend the next week paying attention to the way their body reacts when they are anxious, angry or when they hurt themselves (examples are given in the next box).

'Next time you feel angry or worried, notice how these feelings are reflected in your body. What happens to your shoulders? To your hands? Your jaw? Your breathing? What other parts of your body are affected? How does this feel? Is it helpful?'

'Have you noticed what happens when you stub your toe? What's the first thing you do? Swear? Hold your toe? Tense up? Hold your breath? What else? Have you noticed that it takes a second before you actually feel pain and you've already tensed up in anticipation? Does holding your breath and tensing help?'

In this way you are already linking together the topics of relaxation, breathing and pain. You can build on this when talking about labour in subsequent classes.

Finally, before beginning any practical work, help people explore their attitudes to relaxation. In most groups, some people are keen users already, whereas others have no experience at all and a few think it weird. Women who are planning to have an epidural or an elective caesarian may think relaxation irrelevant. One or two may think that if they learn to relax well they won't feel any pain in labour. Good open questions (see Chapter 9) will involve everyone and help them explore the advantages and limitations of relaxation.

Key points for leading relaxation

Whatever approach you use, the following suggestions can help to make the sessions go well:

- Model a relaxed and unhurried approach. A brisk, businesslike manner is unlikely to put people at their ease.
- In the first session, tension can be reduced by acknowledging that it is strange and perhaps difficult to come into an unfamiliar place, be surrounded by strangers and then be asked to let down one's guard and relax.
- Make the environment as peaceful as possible. Reduce bright lighting and keep noise and interruptions to a minimum. However, if these do occur it's worth pointing out when they happen that labour wards are not always quiet and that being able to relax with activity around will be useful.
- Encourage people to get comfortable and to take their own time to do this. Many people feel they have to keep quite still during a relaxation exercise and despite being very uncomfortable are too embarrassed to move. They certainly won't learn much about relaxation in these circumstances. Invite people to change positions during the session if you notice that anyone looks uncomfortable.
- Think about the positions you suggest people adopt. Do women really need to lie down? Would it be more relevant to encourage them to be more upright?
- Make sure that your voice sounds relaxed. Speak clearly and check that you can be heard by everyone. Remember that you are much more likely to go too fast than to slow – *you cannot talk too slowly when leading relaxation sessions!* Leave pauses between phrases. Although they are familiar to you, they are new to the parents who need time to think and act on what you are saying. Doing the relaxation yourself at the same time (without losing the ability to lead the session!) will help you to get the pace right.
- Choose your words carefully. Use everyday language and develop a whole range of words that conjure up positive images to help

people let go and relax. For example, 'warm', 'soft', 'heavy', 'peaceful', 'open', 'loose'.
- Giggling and laughter are ways people release embarrassment. If you allow them, things will work better in the long run than they would if you try to avoid or suppress them.
- Encourage people to yawn if they feel like it. It does not mean they are bored. It is an excellent way of releasing tension.
- Mention that some women may feel their babies becoming more active as they relax. By suggesting that the babies benefit and enjoy it when their mothers relax, you begin to encourage parents to see their baby as a responsive and sensitive individual.
- End the session gradually. Encourage people to start by becoming aware of their surroundings, then to move slowly and maybe stretch and yawn.
- Afterwards, invite people to review the session by asking some open questions: 'What was that like? What did you enjoy? Find helpful? What was hard? What did you notice about yourself?' This will help people to think about what they experienced and at the same time, give you some useful feedback.

Various methods of relaxation

There is a whole variety of ways to teach relaxation. If you use several throughout the antenatal course, people can experience different ways of relaxing and choose whatever appeals to them most. Because there is no single approach that suits everyone, you will only help the same few people if you use the same approach throughout your course. Choices include:

- contrasting tension with relaxation;
- linking relaxation to breathing;
- linking relaxation to posture and position;
- touch relaxation;
- quick relaxation techniques;
- visualization.

Contrasting tension with relaxation

This method is good as a first introduction, especially if you choose words that really focus people's attention on the difference between relaxation and tension. It helps them recognize what's happening in their bodies and grasp what it feels like to relax. It will take time to do and will require several repetitions during which people's awareness of their bodies and their depth of relaxation increases. You will find one approach to this method in *Simple Relaxation* by Laura Mitchell (see Further Reading at the end of Part II).

Linking relaxation to breathing

Breathing and relaxation are often talked about as separate skills, but in reality they are closely interlinked. It is very hard to let your breathing flow without being relaxed and hard to relax if your breathing is tense and controlled. Linking the two enables people to enhance their awareness and skill in using both to help themselves in labour and to ease the day-to-day stresses of life.

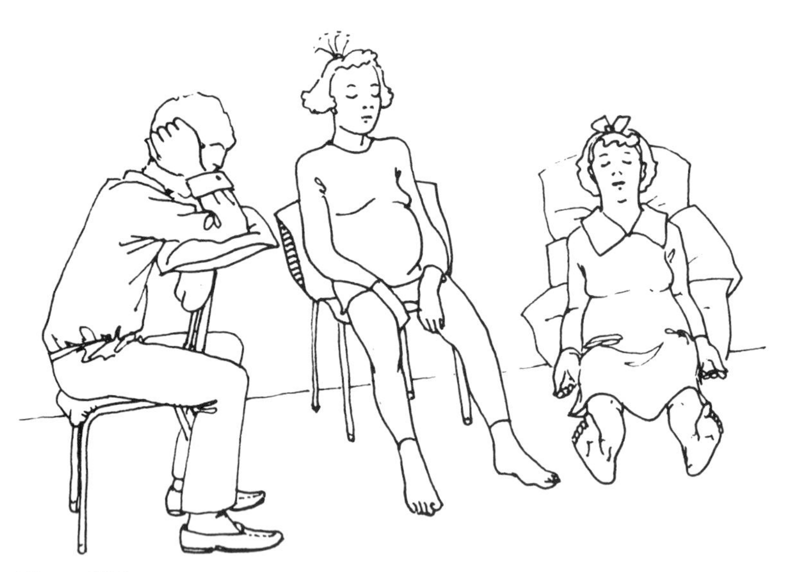

Figure 12.1

You can combine the two approaches just cited. For example, once you have led an initial discussion and helped people to get comfortable, you might begin a first session along the following lines shown in the box (the dots are to remind you to go slowly).

> 'Turn your attention away from the room . . . and towards yourself. Make yourself really comfortable . . . shift about till you've got it just right. . . . Be aware that it isn't always easy to let go in a strange environment with people you don't really know . . . it is fine to take time to get used to it. Let your breathing slow down so that it is gentle and easy . . . and let your breath sigh out every time you breath out. . . . Now I'm going to ask you to pay attention to various parts of your body . . . to tighten them and then let go. First think about your shoulders. . . . Now pull them down towards your feet . . . notice where you feel the tension . . . perhaps down into the tops of your arms? . . . into the centre of your upper back and neck? . . . Really pay attention to how it feels . . . then, as you breathe out, let the tension flow out with your outward breath . . . then notice how your shoulders feel. . . . Try it again, pull your shoulders down . . . feel the tension . . . and breathe it out. Let your shoulders rest . . . feel the difference. . . . (And so on.)

Limiting relaxation to posture and position

Many women will be mobile for the early part of their labour and some will want to be upright and moving about right the way through. Relaxation sessions standing up, sitting or leaning on their partners will prepare women to relax in whatever position they choose. This will also reinforce the message that relaxation is useful throughout life and in a whole variety of situations – sitting on the bus, standing in a queue, at stressful meetings and so on.

In order to help people relax standing up, you need to think carefully about the instructions you give. The instructions given in the box are a basis for you to adapt and use in ways that are comfortable for you and appropriate for the people you teach. Remember to keep the pace slow.

Touch relaxation

This is an excellent way to actively involve partners or encourage women to work together in pairs. It offers women opportunities to

'Stand and find a space where you have room around you . . . it's easier to do this if you take off your shoes. . . . Turn your attention away from the room and towards yourself . . . you may find it better to keep your eyes open so that you don't lose your balance. Just allow your gaze to rest gently on something across the room. . . . Place your feet hip-width apart with your weight equally balanced, so that you have a stable base. . . . Notice your feet in contact with the floor . . . now shift your weight gently onto your toes . . . rock slightly back on your heels . . . shift your weight slightly onto the outside edges of your feet . . . now on the inside edges. . . . Then find a position midway between those four . . . so that you feel evenly balanced . . . in firm contact with the floor . . . you've really got your feet on the ground!

'Now think about your legs . . . bend your knees slightly to ensure they are not locked tightly back . . . breathe out as much tension as you can from your calves and thighs, so that from your hips to your heels your legs feel loose, at ease and comfortable whilst they support you . . . breathe out any tension in your buttocks . . . in the muscles between your legs. . . . Rock your pelvis gently from side to side . . . front to back, circling like a belly-dancer . . . now find a position where your bottom is tucked under, tummy tucked in . . . and the curve in your lower back is reduced. . . . Let your body weight, and for the women, the weight of the baby, be transmitted through your hips into your legs and down to your feet . . . which are firmly in contact with the ground. . . . Let your chest and tummy rise and fall gently and easily with your breathing. . . . Think about your back . . . imagine that you are a puppet and someone is gently pulling the string at the top of your head. . . . Straighten up your body . . . then breathe out and relax without losing the space you have created in your chest and in between each of the little bones in your back. . . . Stand tall . . . relaxed . . . and easy.

'Now drop your shoulders . . . breathe out any tension in your arms . . . let them hang loose and heavy . . . stretch out your fingers and then let them go. . . . Think about your head and neck. . . . Your head weighs around 12 pounds which is a lot to carry around . . . move your head gently from side to side . . . look up . . . down . . . tilt it first to one side . . . then the other. Now find a position midway in between in which your head is lightly balanced on your neck and shoulders . . . imagine your throat getting slightly wider . . . relax the muscles at the back of your neck. . . . Let go of your jaw muscles, let your cheeks be soft and smooth, tongue resting loose in your mouth . . . forehead smooth . . . eyes gazing idly into the distance.

'Now check round your body for any tension and breathe it out. . . . Just enjoy the feeling of being calm and relaxed . . . then, in your own time, start to turn your attention back into the room . . . become more aware of your surroundings, slowly stretch and maybe yawn. . . .'

learn how to relax while they are being touched and while people are moving around them, something that will be part of their experience in labour. It is also a good way to introduce touch into the class, as described in Chapter 13.

Touch involves one person placing his or her hands gently and firmly on a partner's body, sometimes just resting the hands to remind the other person she is not alone. Sometimes, touch includes stroking tension away, usually from the centre to the periphery. The recipient is encouraged to relax towards the hands and to imagine their tension flowing out and away. You will find detailed information on touch relaxation in *The Experience of Childbirth* by Sheila Kitzinger (see Further Reading at the end of Part II).

Quick relaxation techniques

In stressful situations and at the beginning of each labour contraction, people need to be able to relax very quickly. Having established some awareness and skill by using the techniques we have covered so far, you can introduce a variety of methods which will help people to switch at will from tense to relaxed muscles.

'Panic stopping' consists of three simple actions:

- Think STOP.
- Push your shoulders DOWN.
- Breathe OUT long and deliberately, letting all the tension flow out with the outward breath.

'*The relaxation ripple*' consists of releasing tension from the top of the head to the tips of the toes in one continuous wave. When you first teach it, ask people to tense up all over, then to release the tension with a long, slow breath out, relaxing from the top of the body down to the toes in the space of that outward breath. Having practised this once or twice, people should not tense up to start with, but continue to practise simply letting go from head to toe with one long, releasing breath out.

Visualization

There is an infinite variety of visualization techniques you can use with people who have begun to develop some skill in relaxation. Before you decide to use visualization, think through what you are trying to achieve and then devise your own script, using words and phrases that you are comfortable with and which are appropriate to the people you teach. Here are a couple of examples that we particularly like and use frequently.

'Getting in touch with the baby'

This exercise can help parents get in touch with their baby very early in the antenatal course and to recognize that he or she is already a sensitive individual. Having completed a relaxation session with people in comfortable positions (not standing up!) you can invite people to do the boxed suggestions with you. This exercise conveys a lot of information about what the baby is like and can do, in a way which includes the parents. Notice that the words are chosen with care to include fathers. If you talk about 'your uterus', he is left out.

Many people find this exercise an emotional experience and a few (usually women who already have children) will cry afterwards. When they talk about why they reacted in this way, they often say they realize how little time and attention they have given their growing baby because the demands of the child/children they already have are so constant. It usually helps if you encourage them to notice that they have now spent time with the new baby. You could also acknowledge that being pregnant and parenting small children at the same time is extremely demanding and that they are doing their very best under difficult circumstances.

'Now turn your attention towards your baby . . . imagine him or her, curled up inside the uterus, safe, warm and comfortable . . . constantly held . . . always at the right temperature . . . rocked by the mother's movements . . . your baby is already able to hear, is already familiar with the sounds within the mother's body . . . with the rhythms of her heart . . . her breathing and the way she moves . . . He or she is also familiar with the rhythms and cadences of the mother's voice and the voices of those close to her . . . If they have heard their father's voice before birth, newborn babies can recognize his as well as their mother's voice . . . Your baby can already dimly perceive light . . . can suck his or her thumb . . . swallow and pee. He or she may already have recognizable times for rest and activity . . . or be specially prone to hiccups . . . Just spend a few minutes with your baby who is growing and preparing for the birth, just as you are . . . Then . . . in your own time . . . turn your attention back towards your body . . . . and to the room . . . take your time. Remember that you can go back and spend time with your baby whenever you choose.'

'The shopping trip'

This exercise is useful towards the end of the course, when people are familiar with relaxation and have already begun to think beyond the birth to being parents. You could use words like those in the next box.

'Sit comfortably, either in a chair or well propped up with cushions and find something – a pillow, a handbag – to hold as if it is your baby. Place the 'baby' on your chest so that he or she can hear your heartbeat and feel the rhythm of your breathing. Hold him or her gently but securely. Imagine that your baby is three weeks old. You have just come back from shopping . . . you are tired . . . you didn't get much sleep last night . . . You have several bags of shopping to put away . . . the kitchen is a bit of a tip . . . and you are anxious to get on, tidy it up and get the evening meal. Your baby is restless and unsettled even though the last feed was less than an hour ago. Take a decision to leave the shopping and the mess ... It will wait. Settle yourself comfortably with your baby ... hold him or her close to you ... slow your breathing ... and with each outward breath ... let go of the tension in your shoulders ... your neck ... let your head rest or find a position in which it is easily and effortlessly balanced on your neck and shoulders. Breathe out the tension in your jaw ... your cheeks ... smooth out your forehead. Let your arms be soft, welcoming and supportive as you gently cradle your baby. Let your chest and tummy rise and fall peacefully as you breathe ...... Allow your back to sink into the supports ... let go of your legs from your hips to your heels. Just take time to rest ... warm ... safe ... protected and protecting ... enjoy the feeling of your baby snuggled against you ... the softness, warmth and smell of his or her skin. Feel the movements he or she makes ... as you relax and feel peaceful, your baby who is very sensitive to your moods and feelings is likely to do so too. Then, when you have rested ... gently stretch and move ... and slowly prepare to get on with whatever needs to be done.'

It helps if you model a good position in which to sit and hold the 'baby'. It is more graphic if you use a realistic doll to demonstrate this such as we describe in Chapter 14 on visual aids (Figure 12.2).

The benefits of learning relaxation extend far beyond labour. By offering this life skill, you help people to deal with the challenge of labour and enable them to use their bodies more awarely for the rest of their lives.

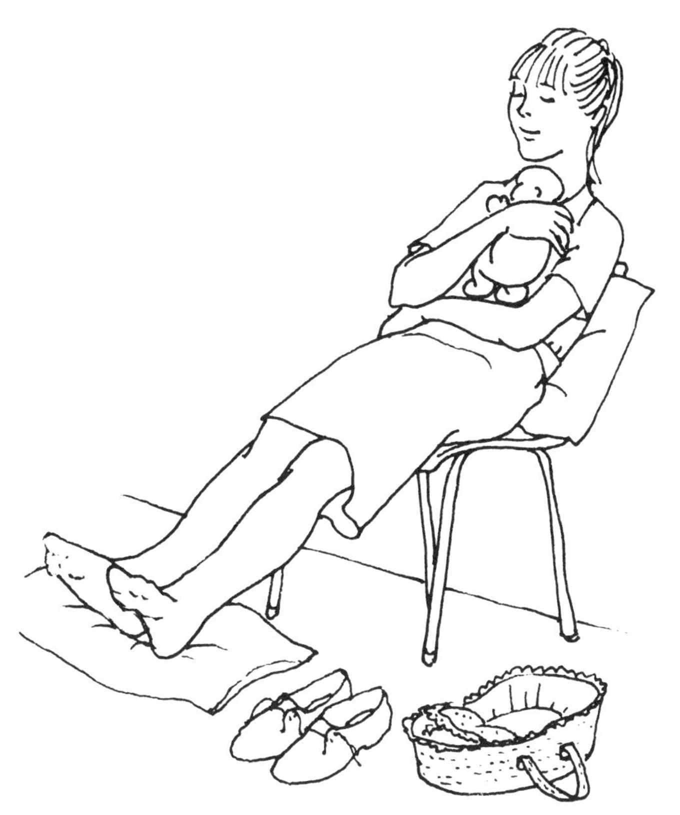

Figure 12.2

13

Breathing, massage, positions and exercise

TEACHING BREATHING

Attitudes to teaching breathing for labour have changed quite dramatically in the past 20 years. At one time, a pattern of defined breathing rates and levels was part of most antenatal teachers' repertoire, whereas now the trend is to encourage women to breathe freely in response to what is happening in their bodies.

Individual antenatal teachers hold convictions anywhere between these two positions. Those who have used imposed patterns in their own labours and found them helpful, often swear by them and communicate their conviction to other women. As a result, some women still say they come to classes to 'learn the breathing', as if mastering this skill will ensure a comfortable, easy labour. Other teachers have seen women try and fail to use breathing patterns so they see little if any benefit in mentioning the topic at all. A few believe teaching breathing to be actually harmful.

As in most matters to do with antenatal education, hard evidence is rarer than firm conviction, so your best option is to examine your own attitudes to discover where you fit on the continuum of structured to *laissez-faire* breathing. What have you read about? What have you seen work? What do women say afterwards about breathing in labour – in the first stage? – at the end of first stage? – in the second stage? If you have given birth, what did you find helpful or unhelpful?

Establishing relevance

Once you have decided how breathing will fit into your course, the next step is to decide how you will teach it. It helps to start by putting breathing into perspective. After all, everyone has managed to breathe through a whole range of painful and stressful experiences. Try asking: 'What happens to your breathing when you climb a long flight of stairs or run for a bus?' This helps people notice that they naturally adapt their breathing when the circumstances demand. You can then focus on issues with relevance to labour by asking: 'What happens to your breathing when you have a pain or stub your toe?' 'When someone gives you a fright?' 'When you are nervous or anxious?'

These questions are likely to elicit the two panic responses seen in labour: over-breathing or breath holding. You can then go on to talk about *and practice* letting one's breathing flow, allowing it to adjust naturally as the stress of the situation demands.

Good practice in teaching breathing

Whatever approaches to breathing you use, the following points may help.

- Model and encourage a relaxed, easy approach.
- Point out that each person is different and will have their own rate and rhythm of breathing both at rest and when under stress.
- Get people to practise. Talking about it is not enough.
- Encourage people to relax more and more deeply with each outward breath even when their breathing is quite rapid.
- Suggest they pause after each outward breath, waiting until their body signals that it is time to let the next breath flow in.
- Choose your words carefully so that they create positive images: 'gentle', 'flowing', 'easy'. Talking about 'slow' breathing rather than 'deep' breathing can help lessen the chances of people hyperventilating.
- Use catchy memorable phrases and imagery. 'If in doubt, breathe out.' Or 'If you get panicky, sigh out and let go like an untied balloon when you release the neck.'
- Explain how to recognize and deal with hyperventilation.

- Encourage feedback and discussion. After practical work, ask what they did and did not find useful. How do they see themselves using what they have done?

Breathing awareness

Through practice, you can help women get in touch with the rates and rhythms they might use in labour and help fathers become familiar with them too. Some find it hard at first. Be especially alert for those who experience difficulty when asked to pay attention to their breathing. They will need extra encouragement to focus on relaxation and let their breathing take care of itself. People in this category often include those with asthma or other conditions in which breathing gets associated with fear and panic, and those who play a brass or wind instrument or sing, all of whom are trained to take a very deep breath and release it slowly and in a very controlled way.

One way to help parents experiment and discover what ways of breathing are available to them is to suggest they sit as in Figure 13.1. Then talk them through a script like the one in the box opposite (the dots are to remind you to go slowly):

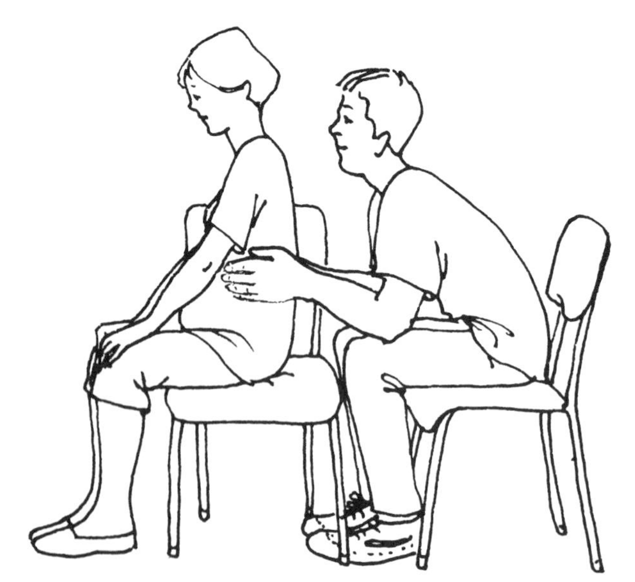

Figure 13.1

'This is an exercise which we'll do just once to help you focus on your ability to adapt your breathing. Let's try it out. If you are sitting at the back, place your hands gently on your partner's waist, or where her waist used to be! Check with your partner they're in the right place. Now the people in front . . . just let your breathing slow down . . . breathe out slowly and gently . . . then pause. Pay attention to your body and when your body tells you it's ready . . . let your breath flow in down towards the hands and then . . . easily and gently . . . sigh out and breathe out any tension . . . then pause until your body signals that it's time to breathe in . . . let it flow in down towards the hands . . . and then sigh out . . . releasing any tension in your shoulders . . . neck . . . jaw. . . . And again, let your breath flow in . . . pause . . . and sigh out, releasing any tension around your body. Just repeat and see if you can establish a rate and rhythm that is comfortable. . . . How does that feel? . . . Anyone light headed? . . . If so, slow down and take it more gently. Really pay attention to waiting until your body wants you to take the next breath in. . . .'

(If it's a couples class) 'It's helpful if the men pay attention to her changing rates and rhythms so that you become familiar with them. Slow gentle breathing is your base-line for labour. It is calming and relaxing . . . it's what fire walkers do for half an hour before walking across hot coals! Some people use it throughout labour . . . others find that as the contractions increase in intensity, they need to change the rate and rhythm. Let's try something different . . . if you're sitting at the back, place your hands in the middle of your partner's back, just let them rest gently. Now, those of you in front . . . just let your breath flow in to the level of the hands . . . then breathe out and pause . . . wait until your body wants you to breathe in again. Notice that your breathing is slightly shallower and a little bit faster.

'Remember to breathe out any tension . . . you can still relax on the outward breath even though your breathing is lighter. Now rest.

Those at the back . . . rest your hands lightly on your partner's shoulders . . . now breathe very softly and gently into the hands, still a slight pause after each out breath, still releasing tension as releasing tension as your breathe out. Find a rate and rhythm that suits you . . . notice that you can breathe quite comfortably at a shallower level and a more rapid rate and still remain calm and relaxed . . . and rest. Now without the hands . . . try out the middle chest breathing again . . . then the slow full breathing and practise changing from one to another. . . . Now change around so your partner gets a chance to try this out and see what it feels like.'

Some teachers offer this awareness exercise, then do no more on breathing *per se*, concentrating instead on increasing parents' skill with relaxation. Other teachers move from being aware of how one is breathing to looking at patterns of breathing appropriate to particular stages of labour.

Linking breathing to changes in labour

Having explained the different rates and rhythms a woman might use during the first stage of labour, you could turn to what might help towards the end of the first stage. Many things can be offered – changing positions, floating in water, a loving companion, making noise, pelvic rocking, general complaining, Entonox, being patient – plus, in some women, a conscious decision to try another way of moving air in and out of their bodies.

Most suggestions for breathing against panic are aimed at both distracting the woman by keeping her brain busy and ensuring her diaphragm keeps moving so that she neither gasps and holds her breath nor bears down before her cervix is open. The easiest ways of doing this are probably the most effective – like sighing out 'Yes . . . yes . . . yes' instead of drawing in breath. Crooning softly to the baby keeps breathing soft, too. Some women want a more ritualized approach, so you might offer them a kind of 'tool kit' of ways from which they might draw should the need arise. It helps if you show several, then ask the women which they prefer *at the moment*, as they may become confused when offered too many choices. Here are some suggestions for teaching anti-panic breathing:

Imagine yourself in a semicircle of candles, all at arm's length. 'One by one, turning your head to face these imaginary candles one by one, just make them flicker. Tiny breaths – don't blow them out – gently, slow, slow. Now, the contraction is fading so breathe slower, sighing out the tension.'

Make your mouth into an O and breathe out gently saying 'Hoo hoo', then make your lips wide and loose, then breathe out again, saying 'Haa, haa'. Pause. Then do it again, slowly, then again. Keep checking that your jaw stays soft. Now the contraction starts to fade so follow the diminishing strength of the contraction with your breath.

Allow your head and shoulders to sway gently to the left and let your breath out. Pause. Then sway gently the other way and let your breath out. Pause. . . . This goes particularly well with moaning, making the kind of round, open-throated noises that let feelings out.

Women will only be able to breathe like this for a short time when in labour. Help them to see how breathing like this is a way of allowing their bodies to work *with* what is happening rather than drawing away from it. When learning these patterns, they will need your help in seeing how they might fit them into the over-all pattern of a contraction.

Modelling contractions

If you think it is useful to link changes in breathing with the pattern of contractions, you will need to find some way of showing what a contraction is like, although you will never replicate the real sensation. One way to give a glimpse of what is coming is to talk them through a contraction, allowing your voice to get louder, faster and more urgent as you describe the increasing strength and tightness of the uterus. You could add external noise to your description, perhaps by turning up the static on an untuned radio as the 'contraction' grows stronger or by shaking a hand-held rattle to mirror its strength. Ask parents to notice how the noise and urgency affect them. Remind them to practise going *with* something they don't like, rather than fighting against it.

Another way to help them link how they are breathing with what their bodies are doing is to suggest they assume a position that usually results in breath holding or tension. Try these yourself before suggesting them to others:

- Kneel up with your bottom tucked in and back straight, then lean the top of your body back slightly. *Be sure to keep your back straight and bottom well tucked under*. What happens when you lean slightly farther back? As you hold the position, what changes do you notice in your tension or breathing over 10 or even 20 seconds?

- Sit on the floor with one leg bent and one leg stretched out then, keeping your back straight, lean towards the outstretched foot. Can you feel the stretch in your inner thighs? What happens to your breath? . . . to your shoulders? . . . to your jaw? What happens when you increase the stretch a bit? Try breathing into the stretch, relaxing and letting go. What happens?

(Chapter 14 carries further suggestions about modelling contractions.)

Breathing for the second stage

For years, women were taught that in the second stage they should fill their lungs, fix their diaphragms and produce as much intra-abdominal pressure as they could for as long as they could. This way of pushing – usually called 'block-and-push' – has little place in an antenatal course because it has been shown to be bad for babies, not much fun for mothers and no more effective than more gentle ways of using one's breathing to help a baby be born. The only use for rigid breathing patterns in the second stage is to teach how to push with an epidural. These women will have no internal signals telling them when and how strongly to bear down. Even here, the old 'block-and-push' technique will need modifying so that women bear down for no more than five or six seconds before snatching a breath. This gives the baby the recovery time he or she needs to cope well with the second stage.

Instead of teaching standard second-stage breathing, you could show them what a woman in labour looks like and sounds like. Show them how she breathes – perhaps with several short, shallow breaths as the contraction begins, then bearing down for a few seconds with an exhalation, letting your breath go and perhaps making a noise as you do so. Show them how in one contraction a woman can bear down two or three times, catching her breath between. Talk about how a pushing urge can be overwhelming and far too strong to ignore. If you are miming the delivery as you talk as suggested in Chapter 14, interrupt yourself in mid-sentence and do another 'contraction' to show how inexorable the process is.

Once group members have a sense of how women might breathe in the second stage, you could encourage them to try it themselves. One way to help them do so is to suggest the woman sits well propped up and that someone else – her partner or another woman if group members know each other well – places a firm hand over her pubic symphysis. Ask the woman to drop her chin, open her mouth loosely, take a few short breaths and see if she can make the hand move with her breath. Encourage her to push towards the hand so that her effort isn't 'stuck' in her neck. She might imagine her breath leaning on the baby's bottom while she relaxes her pelvic floor to let the baby out.

Improving your own skills

If you are still developing your own approach to teaching breathing, you will probably need to collect other people's ideas and try them out yourself. You will find many suggestions in Further Reading at the end of Part II. Talk with colleagues about what they do and why they feel it works. Keep your eyes open for study days advertised in the professional journals or run by voluntary organizations like those listed in Appendix I. Above all, listen to parents. Their postnatal feedback will be your best guide to shaping whatever you do with breathing. That, plus your own attitudes and convictions, will help you fashion an approach to breathing that works for the women you teach and feels right for you.

TEACHING MASSAGE

Touch is increasingly being rediscovered as being therapeutic. It eases the physical and emotional stresses of everyday life and the special aches and pains of pregnancy and labour. Touching helps couples express affection and communicate with each other and with their baby once he or she is born. There are many different ways you can encourage aware, helpful touch and massage in an antenatal course. You could teach touch relaxation; self-massage; strong back or thigh massage; perineal massage; effleurage; foot massage; or baby massage. There is a variety of books which decribe these and other techniques (see Further Reading at the end of Part II).

Individual antenatal teachers vary enormously in what they think useful and appropriate when it comes to massage. Many are hesitant and self-conscious about the topic, a surprising attitude when you consider the intimate ways in which midwives, in particular, touch their clients. However, health professionals are trained to touch in ritualized ways and with a degree of detachment. There are good reasons for this and it works well for many procedures. But therapeutic touch (touch that helps the other person feel better) requires greater involvement from the person doing the touching. That is something that health professionals have been encouraged to avoid.

How do you feel about teaching massage? What other factors will sway your choices as to what to include or omit? One way to find out is to talk with a supportive colleague. If inexperience is a factor, you could ask a friend to work with you, giving and receiving a whole range of techniques including some that don't immediately appeal to you. Tell each other what you each enjoyed receiving and what the giver did well. If you get the chance, attend a workshop or study day on massage. Then reconsider what you will include in your course.

Fitting massage into your course

The next step is to think about where in the course massage will fit, so that it links in with other topics under consideration. A gradual introduction usually works best, moving from safe to more intimate ways of touching. If the group is new or has many shy members, introduce touch relaxation or back massage, linking it to learning to relax. That's something most people expect to learn in classes. Once the group is comfortable, short massage sessions can be interspersed as a break from other activities or, when appropriate, used to change the atmosphere.

However sensitively you approach massage, expect some self-consciousness and embarrassment. Our society conditions many of us (and men in particular) to believe that touch is only relevant as a precursor to sex, so touching in public will seem odd. It helps if you begin by talking about 'touch' rather than 'massage', which for some has a rather dubious reputation. Be sensitive to the needs of the group. Some religions and cultures forbid touching between the sexes in public, so check with the people you are teaching and when necessary, find ways of introducing it which allow some people not to participate.

Good practice in teaching massage

Whatever type of massage you teach, the following can help to make the session go well.

- Make sure everyone has someone to work with.
- Invite someone who you think will be willing to be demonstrated on. Show people, step by step, what you suggest they try.
- Model a relaxed, confident approach which focuses on and completely respects the person you are touching.
- Invite people to do it themselves, coaching them step by step in the beginning.
- If you are working with a mixed group of men and women, you could suggest that women try it on their partners first. Women have usually received less conditioning than men and are often freer to touch with sensitivity. The men will then have an opportunity to learn, by receiving, what feels good and are likely to feel less self-conscious and threatened when roles are reversed.
- Suggest the touchers shake out their hands so they are relaxed and then let their hands mould to the shape of the part they are touching.
- Make sure that the person doing the massage is comfortable. This is a good time to point out that being a labour companion is tiring and that men need to conserve their energy too! Pay particular attention to the partner's back and be alert for straining.
- Don't be put off by laughter and giggling – it's a good way for people to release their embarrassment. Remind them that everyone in the room is concentrating on what they are doing and that nobody is being watched.
- Encourage recipients to tell their partner what feels good, rather than criticizing. For example, 'It feels wonderfully relaxing on my legs, and it would be great if you could use more pressure over my feet; they're ticklish.' This confirms the person doing the touching in his or her skills instead of feeling 'I got it wrong', and offers constructive information for doing it differently.

- Instead of telling parents they are doing something wrong, demonstrate an alternative and support them in trying it out.
- Afterwards, ask the group to review the experience. What did they like? What might be useful in labour? In everyday life? When they or their partners are tired or stressed? What do they think their baby might enjoy?

Often, following a massage session, the group is relaxed and ready to receive some information or engage in real discussion. You could suggest that touch is a lovely way to show each other affection without having sex, something that may not be welcomed by some women towards the end of pregnancy or in the early days after the birth. You can also point out that babies love to be touched and that by practising touching each other awarely they are learning a skill that their baby will very much appreciate. In this way, a teacher uses the experience of shared massage to build a safe, supportive group from a cluster of individuals.

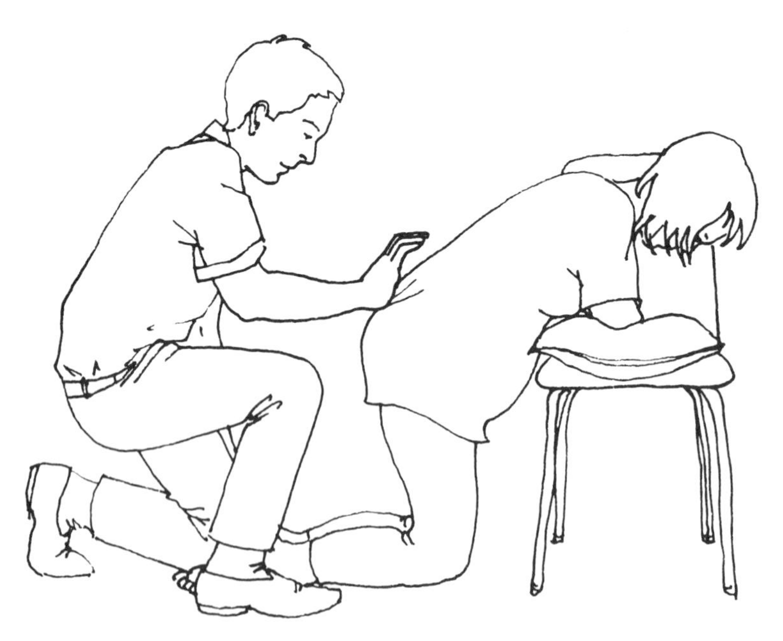

Figure 13.2

TEACHING POSITIONS

Teaching positions for labour

Claims for the clinical benefits of upright posture and mobility in labour continue to be hotly debated, but the evidence in favour grows ever more persuasive. Whatever the merits of the arguments pro and con, there is no doubt that many women feel better emotionally as well as physically if their head is literally as well as metaphorically above their uterus. Most women will be upright for at least part of their labour and a number remain so right the way through. By helping people discover a variety of positions and offering them opportunities to link these with relaxation, you equip them to respond flexibly in labour.

As usual, your own experience and attitudes are important. Whatever you say or do, your true feelings will be evident to the people you teach. Assess your opinions by considering the questions in the box. Talking through your opinions and listening attentively to others, especially those with different views and experiences from your own, can help you to keep a balanced perspective.

- How do you feel about women being active and mobile throughout labour?
- Do you think it unnecessary?
- Is it too inconvenient for those trying to monitor the baby and care for the mother?
- Can it be dangerous?
- What benefits have you seen or experienced?
- What clinical advantages might there be?
- What do women who have remained mobile throughout labour tell you?

Once you are clear about your views on the relevance of positions to labour, share your conclusions with parents lest they see practising positions as nothing more than a strange series of contortions. You might put the whole issue into an historical perspective, pointing out that women throughout the world and throughout the ages have adopted a variety of positions for labour and delivery. One way to focus people's attention on the issue of positions is to tell the apocryphal tale about King Louis XIV liking to watch babies being born, a proclivity that meant the woman had to lie down so he got a good view. The supine position was apparently then justified as being the 'modern' way to give birth!

Now, the opposite is true. You can show parents why this is so by demonstrating the passage that the baby takes through the birth canal or by holding charts or a doll and pelvis in various positions to make the differences come to life. As you move a pelvis from horizontal to upright postures, they can see how the mobility of the sacrum is lost if the mother's weight is on her lower back. You can talk about the benefits of gravity and the advantages of not having the weight of the uterus pressing on the mother's main blood vessels in both the first and second stages.

Your discussions should also focus on ways of adapting the labour room to accommodate various positions by moving furniture, clearing a floor space, or bringing items like cushions or a child's small step stool from home. Equally, parents may need to adapt themselves and their positions to accommodate the surroundings, choosing positions to suit labour at home, in the car, when an epidural is in place, or in a very public ward (Figures 13.3–13.9).

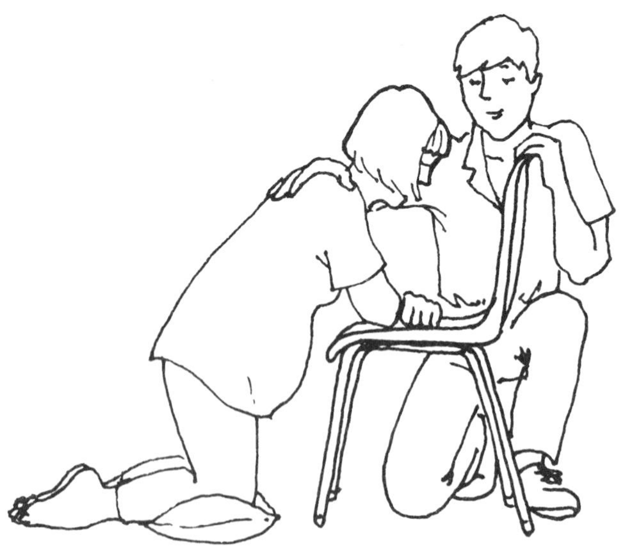

Figure 13.3

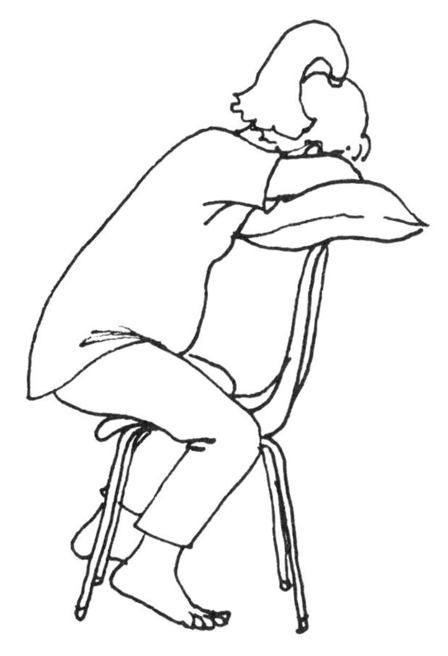

Figure 13.4

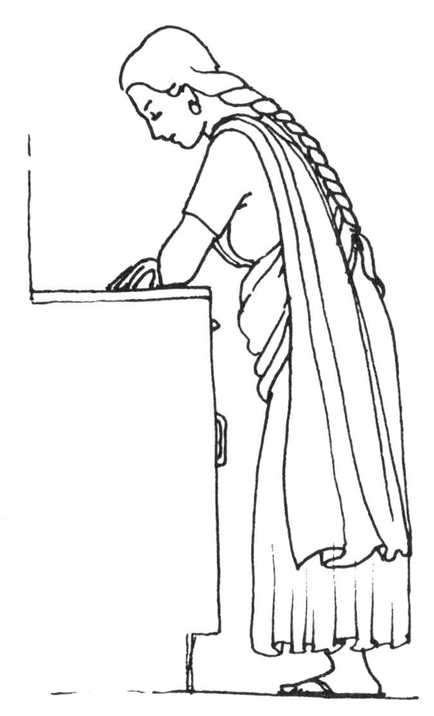

Figure 13.5

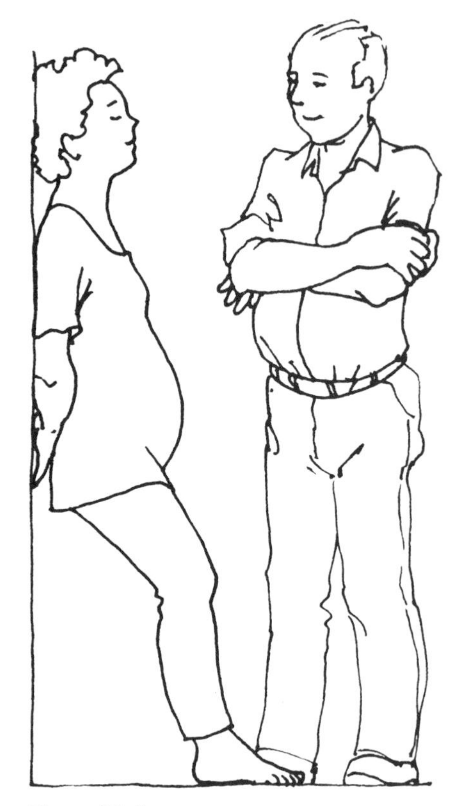

Figure 13.6

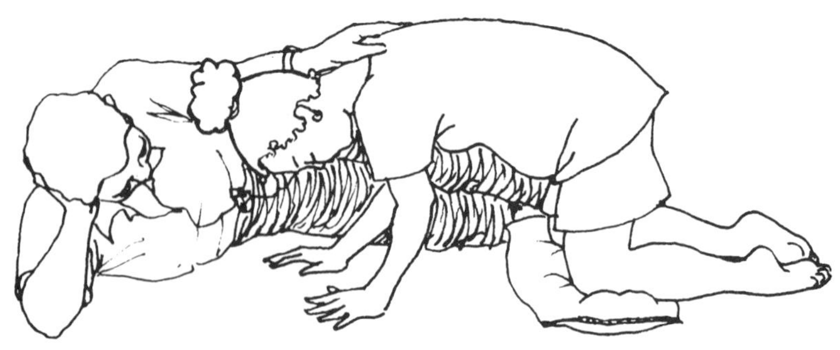

Figure 13.7

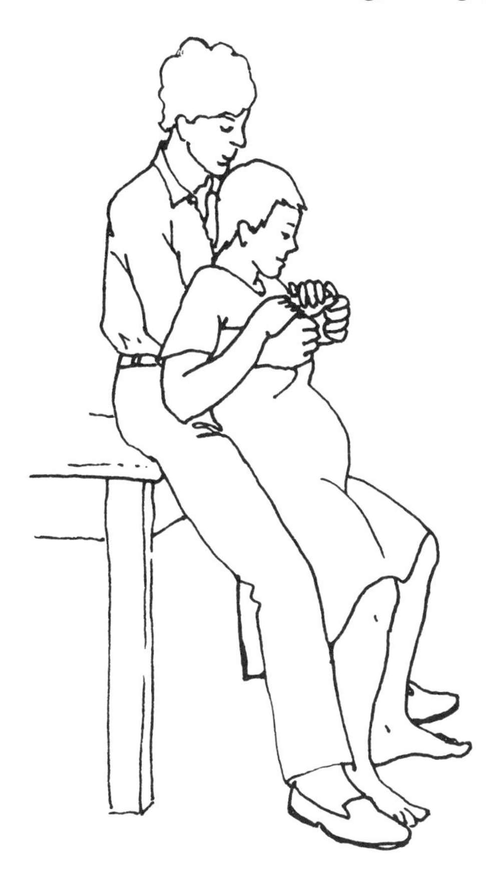

Figure 13.8

Here are some key points for teaching positions in labour:

- Keep your information-giving short and spend the maximum amount of time on practice.
- Suggest that people wear loose, comfortable clothing to classes and do the same yourself. Negotiate with your superiors if wearing a uniform is the norm – does this have to be so? Many professionals have changed this custom and find there are more benefits than just the ease of teaching positions.
- Use a relaxed, casual approach when demonstrating.
- Be determined and persuasive about getting people going. Acknowledge their reluctance or lethargy, but keep up your cheerful chivvying until they move.

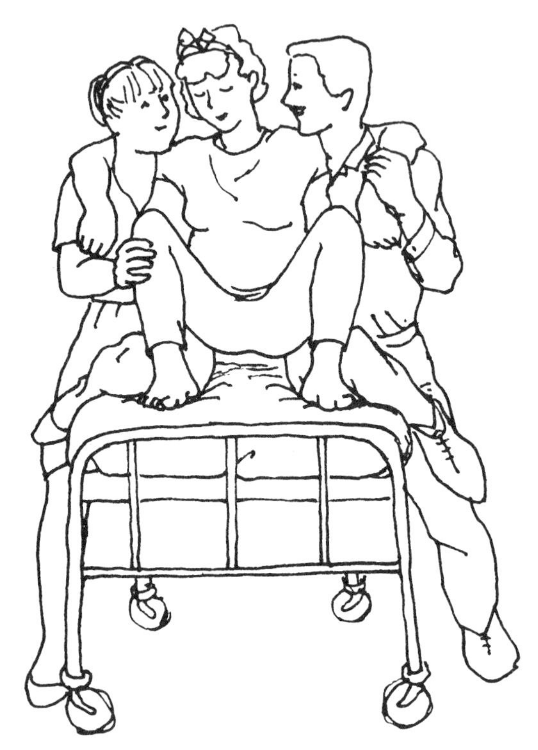

Figure 13.9

- Encourage people to try out and practise a variety of positions. What they like and dislike now, may not apply in labour. What suits early first stage, may not work later on in labour.
- Encourage parents to keep trying new positions in labour. Just as turning over into a new position during a sleepless night can help, changing positions during labour can in itself make things more tolerable.
- Build in opportunities for practice throughout the course.
- Link practice of positions to relaxation, breathing awareness or massage.
- Encourage people to experiment at home: Which bits of furniture are the right height to lean on? Do you have a chair to sit on back-to-front? How would you be comfortable travelling in a car?
- If you are teaching couples, encourage the men to help their partners get comfortable in a variety of positions.

TEACHING EXERCISE

Research data do not support the idea that fitter women have easier births. However, they do show that anyone, pregnant or non-pregnant, benefits from moderate exercise as long as it is done three or more times a week and is supervised by skilled people. Benefits for pregnant women from regular exercise include suppleness and better endurance to help a mother feel better; stronger muscles to cope with changes in posture and to decrease the discomforts of pregnancy; and continuity with a woman's former non-pregnant lifestyle.

Women who cannot or decide *not* to devote time and effort to fitness during pregnancy can be helped to see that they are not putting themselves or their babies at increased risk. Of course, women who neglect fitness will miss out on the benefits of regular exercise listed above.

In a course which balances the three elements mentioned in Chapter 5 – information sharing, discussion and physical skills – the focus will be on teaching people new ways to use their bodies, rather than helping them get fit for labour. Parents need to know this before they come or early in the first session, lest they expect a workout. Of course, should they want more vigorous exercises, there are plenty of classes, books and tapes teaching fitness for pregnant women. In most of them, the teacher probably believes that energetic preparation will improve a woman's chances of getting the birth she wants. That's an idea many parents find attractive, despite the lack of evidence showing fitness to be an influence on labour. Unless you tell them what kind of class you are running, they could be disappointed if your approach is not particularly vigorous.

So if you don't teach exercises for fitness, what do you teach? We opt for three exercises that involve muscles directly connected with pregnancy and birth : pelvic floor exercises, pelvic rocking/tilting, and tailor-sitting or other ways of stretching the inner thighs. These three have the added advantage of jiggling the inhibitions as much as the muscles themselves! Ways to improve posture are also helpful for some women, although very few put them into long-term use.

Pelvic floor exercises

When teaching pelvic floor exercises, it is best to begin early in the course because most women feel little or no reaction to their efforts for several weeks. Most antenatal teachers use analogies to get across what they want – lifts, drawbridges, making love, even keeping a tampon in place. Make sure you choose ones that feel appropriate for you and be aware that parents may find some more acceptable than others. If women have no idea where the muscles are to which you are referring, ask them to blow sharply into a fist. This usually produces a 'kick' in the appropriate place that most can feel. Some women cannot isolate muscles around their vaginas and benefit from doing pelvic floor exercises while sitting on their hands, an easy way to feel buttocks tightening.

Most pregnant women have a hard time remembering to practise and will need frequent reminders. 'Few and often' usually works best, perhaps linking practice to everyday activities like standing at the sink or getting up from the sofa. As the weeks pass, you will need to enquire regularly as to their progress and reassure them that they will soon be exercising more than their eyebrows! And by the way, since this really is a skill for life, when was the last time *you* did pelvic floor exercises for your own benefit?

Pelvic rocking/tilting

These exercises are good ways to get women moving about and trying things out once you have discussed their use in maintaining mobility, relieving backache during pregnancy and helping in labour. They are fairly non-threatening and the skills themselves are easy to learn. If you wish, you can also provoke giggling by encouraging belly-dancing or other unusual movements and, in the process, subtly change how the group works together. Pelvic rocking and tilting is also an ideal way, anywhere in a course, to give the group a five-minute energy boost. Use it whenever you feel the group needs to move, get their circulation going or recover from a gloomy discussion.

Other physical skills

You will doubtless come across many more physical skills as you keep your eyes and ears open, read books and listen to women postnatally. Part IV includes strategies for helping you plan how you will incorporate new skills into your course.

14

Visual aids

Good visual aids enhance information giving and entertain. They bring into the antenatal class the sights, sounds and experiences of the outside world and make real the hidden world within the body. Although called *visual* aids, this chapter looks at ways to actively involve other senses like sound and touch as well as sight.

As you read this section, you may think, That sounds complicated. This is because verbal descriptions very often are complicated and long-winded compared with a 'look at this' explanation – proof that a picture is worth a thousand words.

Using your own body

The best visual aid you have is yourself. Whatever you *say*, your voice, gestures and actions will reveal how you *really* feel. Using your body expressively and imaginatively will help parents grasp and remember the concepts you introduce. You could do this by any of the following methods.

Illustrating on yourself

When using posters or photographs, link what is shown to your own body. For example:

- stand sideways to match cross-section drawings;
- hold life size charts up against you;
- show the length and location of a caesarian scar with a neat, small gesture on your own body;
- show where your diaphragm, coccyx, pubic symphysis and pelvic brim are, then encourage parents to find theirs;

- hold the doll up against your own body to show lie and engagement.

Demonstrating an action

If you want parents to master a skill, they will need practice and participation. If your demonstration is to enhance understanding, it will help them remember if you make your actions as realistic as possible. Thus, when you are showing how to get back in bed after a caesarian section, demonstrate the effort and discomfort (and don't forget to breathe out and drop your shoulders when it 'hurts' . . .).

Miming

Many common procedures are easily adapted to mimes. Your cupped hands can become two forceps blades. Place a doll in front of you, feet facing away, then winkle your right cupped hand along the left side of the doll's head, copying the usual actions of whoever is applying the forceps. Do the same with your left hand along the right side of the doll's face (note that your hands are now crossed) and 'lock' your elbows. You can then pull appropriately while talking parents through the procedure.

Showing what not *to do*

Demonstrations are particularly useful for showing what *not* to do – how *not* to stand or lift or rub a woman's back. Exaggerating your 'mistakes' will make parents feel less anxious because no matter how amateur their own effort, it is bound to be better than what they have just seen!

Modelling something invisible

Many of the things antenatal teachers describe are hidden or secret. By creating something similar, you offer parents an image they can understand.

- As you talk, your tight fist may 'become' a cervix '(Figure 14.1).
- In another context, push your thumb between the second and third fingers of your clenched fist, and you have a satisfactory 'nipple' (Figure 14.2).

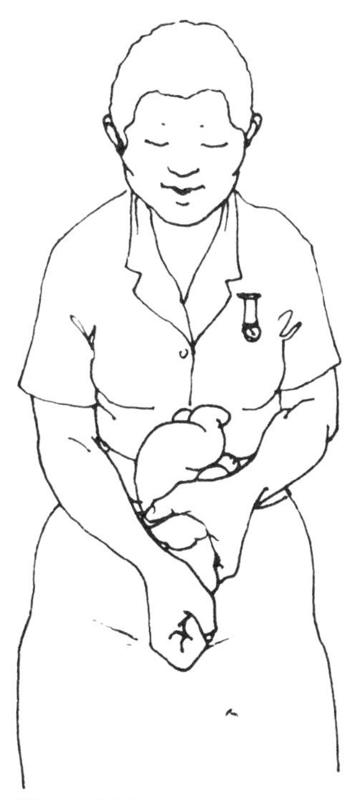

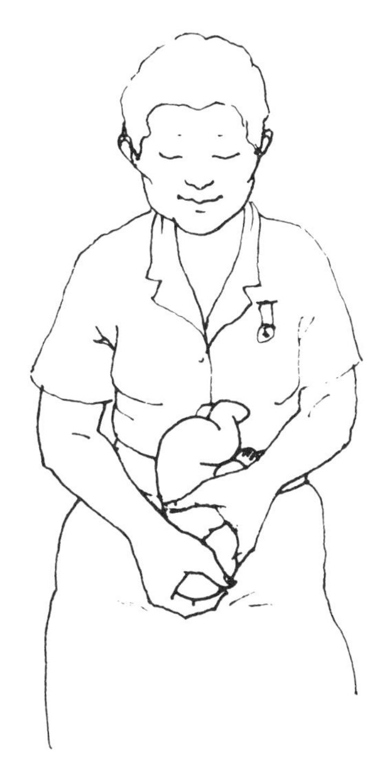

Figure 14.1

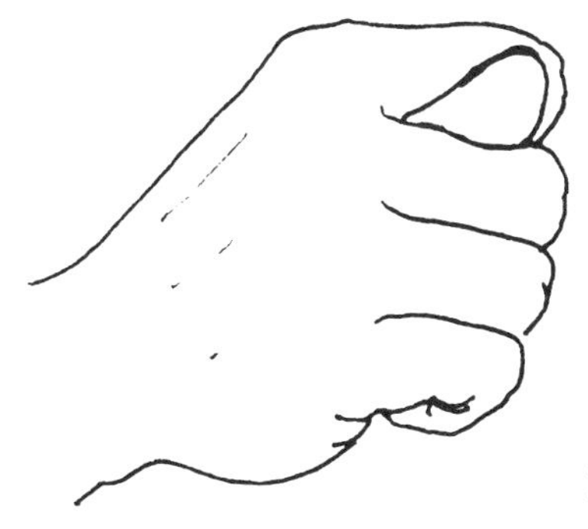

Figure 14.2

- Two hands gradually drawing back over your bowed head until they rest around your ears will translate dilatation from an abstract notion to something real and tangible (Figure 14.3).
- Or stretch wide your thumb and first finger until you see the arch of skin between them, then talk about an 'anterior lip' with your other

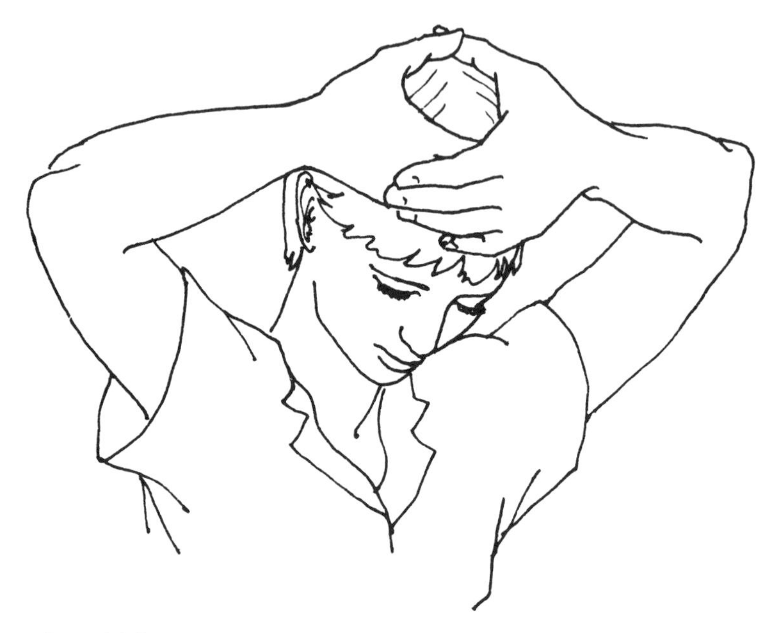

Figure 14.3

hand making a fist for the baby's head. Alternatively, the same flap can help parents understand an episiotomy. Point thumb and fingers upward, draw a round circle in the appropriate place below the arch of skin for an 'anus' then, while you talk about the procedure, add a J-shaped line to show where and how long an episiotomy might be (Figure 14.4).

You can even model the whole of the first stage. Ask the group to each make two fists and put them together, knuckle to knuckle, over their pubic bone (Figure 14.5). Say something like, 'Now look down – your arms represent the sides of a uterus and the fists a tightly closed cervix. See the gap between your knucles? That's like the passage your baby will go through.' Ask them to 'half-uncurl' their fists and place bent fingers together, then talk about effacement. Next, put finger tip to finger tip: 'Still no way through yet for your baby but the cervix is ready to open.' Now's the time to mention the latent phase of labour. . . . Then encourage them to slowly open the way, bit by bit to 10 centimetres.

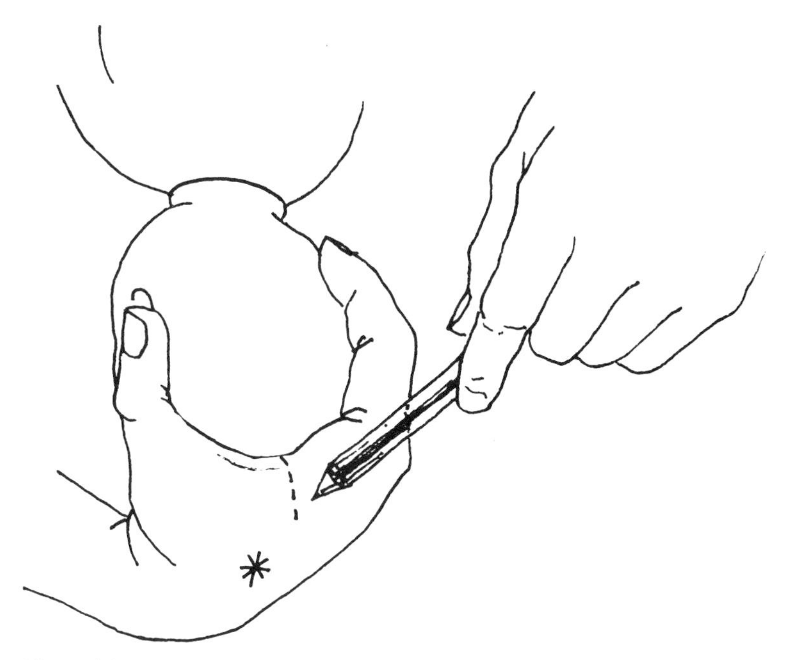

Figure 14.4

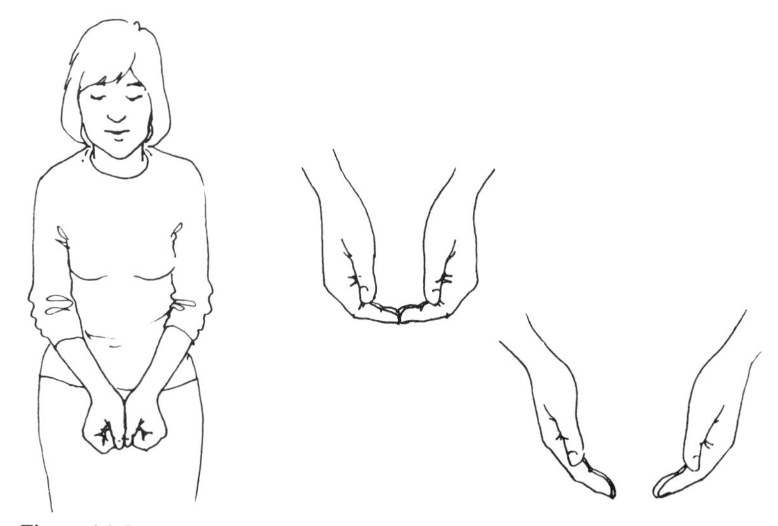

Figure 14.5

We have done this sequence with large groups, carefully choosing words applicable to both men and women. The whole room becomes breathless with excitement as they 'see' the sequence actually happening. (As a variation, ask them to do 'dilatation' again in pairs, with one person being the 'midwife', assessing the gap with his or her eyes closed.)

As well as sights, you can model sensations. Put your fingers in both corners of your mouth and pull gently. Feel the stretch? Then a bit harder . . . and a bit harder! Usually, people describe their lips as hot and tingly; some mention pain and fear; most say their lips feel numb and cold when they let go. The parallels with crowning are obvious and enlightening.

Acting

Once parents understand the mechanics of a contraction, you can paint a more realistic picture by adding the sounds of labour. Try a groan, whimper slightly, catch your breath with a sharp pain then breathe out, drop your shoulders and let the contraction happen. Add the look of labour by turning your attention away from the room, dropping your head, rocking from side to side, shifting position and leaning on the person next to you – whatever you feel is realistic, ordinary behaviour for a woman in labour.

Alternatively you can invite class members to try out simulated contractions in which they experience some of the tension and discomfort. There is a variety of ways you can choose from although it is important to stress that they will not experience how contractions actually feel but will gain some idea of how they might react.

As you talk the class through a timed contraction, increase the volume of your voice, adding tension and desperation into your tone as the contraction reaches its peak, then become quieter and calmer as it wanes.

You can ask people to try any of the following and to hold it, relax and breathe through the discomfort:

- clutch an ice cube as tightly as possible; *or*
- kneel with knees apart, then lean back till there is a stretch in the thighs; *or*
- stand with their back to the wall and slide down keeping their back supported until their knees are slightly bent and they feel tension in their thighs.

We would encourage anyone to develop their acting ability, perhaps saving the sounds of pain and panic until group members feel comfortable with each other and the teacher has a sense of what will and will not work. You will probably discover, as we have, that parents identify so closely with what you are doing that they actually believe they are witnessing the real thing and get a glimpse of how they might feel and react.

However, the idea of doing a realistic demonstration of a contraction often startles health professionals, especially those for whom this kind of extrovert behaviour is out of character. If you feel this way, could you start with other mimes? Show them the quick-breathing, head-waving search of a newborn looking for the nipple or the cautious way a woman with stitches sits down.

Visual aid equipment

The teaching doll

After your own body, a teaching doll is the most important tool you have when working with parents. It may take some effort to find the ideal teaching doll, but it will be time well spent.

A good doll must be attractive. Look for a face you find pretty, a well-shaped body and, bearing in mind the people you teach, choose a cloth doll with a skin colouring they could identify with. Your doll needs to be nearly the same size as a newborn baby and flexible to the elbows and knees. It should also feel right when you cuddle it. If you teach by putting your doll through a model pelvis, make sure it goes without shoving or getting stuck. (We have always found shopkeepers helpful but quizzical when we take the pelvis along to the shop and test possible dolls before purchase.) When you have the doll home, unpick a seam and take out a third or more of the stuffing for a suitably floppy feel.

Always treat your doll like a real baby. Wrap it in a shawl, keep it tucked up in a padded box or other carrying case, and wash it and its blankets regularly to keep them pristine. When you handle your doll, talk to it and apologize for any awkward manoeuvres. Make sure you cradle its head when you wrap and unwrap it and put it back gently when you are finished. In this way, you are not only helping parents visualize their own baby, you are teaching parentcraft skills. This may be the first time that some parents have seen a 'baby' held with love, comforted, winded. . . . . For most observers, within seconds your teaching doll *is* their baby. Their gasp of horror should you forget and handle the doll roughly or fling it into its box will be proof of their identification.

Hand-made aids

Apart from a knitted uterus (although we both prefer using a child's striped jersey with extra elastic in the polo neck), there is a host of useful things that even the most unhandy person can make.

A placenta

Cover a dinner plate sized piece of one-inch thick sponge rubber with dark red material such as towelling (the knobblier the better.)

An umbilical cord

Buy three metre-long lengths of thick cord from a drapers shop (dressing gown cord or the kind you use to tie back heavy curtains). One of the lengths should be scarlet, the other two darker red or purplish to mimic veins and arteries. Twist the lengths together and fix the twist by tacking with needle and thread. Then, on one end of the twisted cord, stitch half a popper, using the other half to make a 'navel' for the doll so the cord can snap on and off. Unravel the other end of the twisted cord and fan the strands out across the surface of your cloth 'placenta'. Once you have found a realistic pattern for these strands, stitch them in place.

Embryos and fetuses

Cut out silhouettes of life-size babies at four weeks gestation (the size of a grain of rice), six weeks (the size of a black-eyed bean), eight weeks (the size of a broad bean) and 12 weeks (the size of a dried fig). Most embryology books contain accurate drawings of fetuses at these ages. Two silhouettes, cut from thick card and glued together, will make a more rounded, realistic 'baby', as will colouring the card pinkish and adding a closed eye in the appropriate place.

Pass these tiny 'babies' (or the above mentioned food items) around, cradling them gently. Invite discussion on what it felt like to hold such a tiny creature and talk about what their babies could do at those stages of growth.

A perineum

Cut a hole in the bottom of a plastic kitchen bowl large enough to fit your doll's head easily. Then cut a circle of thin foam rubber larger than the hole and lay it in the bottom of the bowl. It will fit better if you glue and shape the foam so it is bowl shaped, too. Cut a cross-shaped opening in the foam rubber big enough to accommodate the doll's head without tearing. When using the contraption, put it between your knees at about the angle of a woman's pelvis.

By pushing against the bottom of the bowl with your doll's head, you can mimic the bulging perineum and crowning head of the end of the second stage. Your actions and noises can make this in some ways realistic. Some antenatal teachers put the doll inside a plastic bag (explaining to the group that this is just for the purpose of the demonstration) as the resulting shiny, wet appearance echoes the membranes.

Others demonstrate crowning and birth by sitting in a semi upright position, placing the doll on their lower abdomen, under a sweater or covered with a blanket and use their hands over the doll's head to demonstrate the two steps forward, one back of the second stage, crowning and delivery. By miming several contractions, adding realistic noises and demonstrating effort, you can simulate a second stage which gives expectant parents a picture not just of the physical aspects of birth but also of the emotional intensity of the experience.

Of course, demonstrating birth in these ways needs practice and demands a sense of humour about your early efforts!

'Found' items

There are endless everyday things that can illustrate and enhance the information you give. Here are some examples.

Balloons

Blow them up full, slap on a lick-and-stick parcel label with 'placenta' written on it, let half the air out and watch the label buckle and detach. It's the ideal beginning to a discussion about what happens in a physiological third stage.

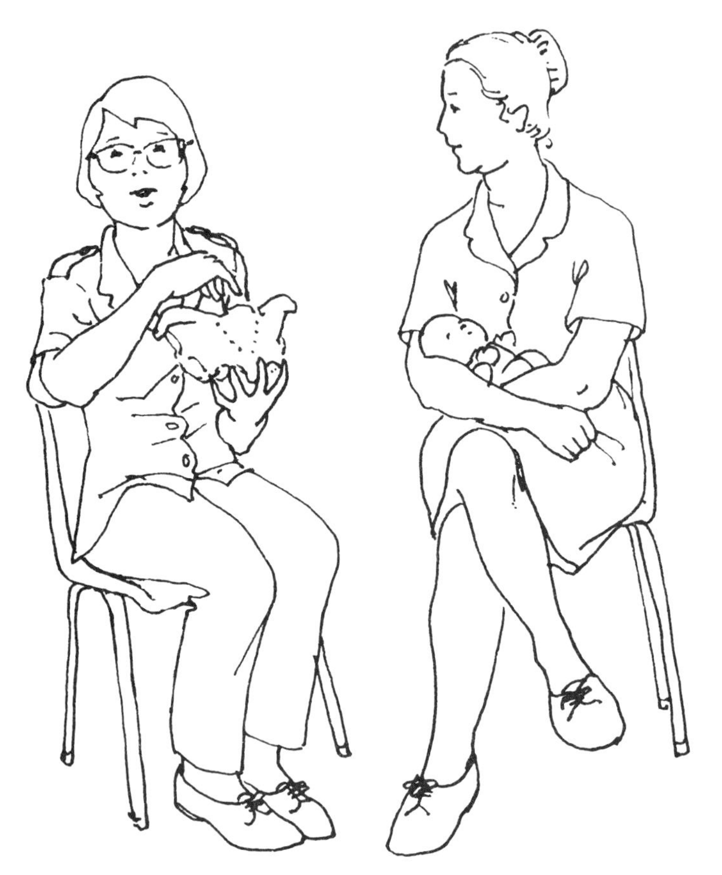

Figure 14.6

Clothes pegs

These make excellent reusable cord clamps.

Fruit

A bunch of grapes illustrates the anatomy of the breast. Bananas demonstrate the curve through which the baby travels during the second stage and give women a picture of the direction in which to push. A pear, cut longitudinally, looks like a just-pregnant uterus.

Drive belt from an upright vacuum cleaner

Useful to demonstrate a fully dilated cervix because most are 10 centimetres across and they are stretchy.

The 'real thing'

Collect and pass round the paraphernalia parents might encounter during their stay in hospital, such as a scalp electrode, amnihook, epidural set-up, Entonox mask, forceps or monitor tracing. You may think of other things that parents find surprising or anxiety-producing. As they touch it, turn it over in their hands and perhaps make nervous jokes about it, their fantasies are slowly reduced to more manageable levels and the mystique around what is, in fact, just a piece of equipment begins to fade. You can also offer them as much hands-on experience as possible during the hospital tour.

You can also use real sounds – tapes of a baby continually crying and crying; a grizzly baby; an actual birth; the first greeting between mother, father and baby; womb sounds; a noisy sucking baby and so on. These can be used on their own or added to relaxation and visualization exercises as appropriate.

Photographs

Photographs of techniques and equipment are almost as good as seeing the real thing. So, too, is a series of photos that tell a story (i.e. the same baby, photographed six or seven times during a feed). Photos should be large, perfectly in focus, clear and modern. If you have no good ones, contact your nearest technical college or suggest a budding sixth-form photographer take a series as a project.

Good photocopying shops will do blow-ups of textbook illustrations and some even have colour facilities. However, you should ensure you do not violate copyright laws. If you want to use a photo more than once, mount it on stiff card and cover it with transparent plastic. Parents will welcome the chance to handle, inspect and pass around the photos themselves. That process is part of their ownership of the information, a process made more difficult if the teacher holds on to everything.

Charts, posters and diagrams

There is a range of charts and diagrams available to antenatal teachers (see Appendix II) or you can devise your own. Here are some points to bear in mind when choosing and using charts and diagrams.

- If you have a set of diagrams or charts, look at them critically and use only those that illustrate the points you want to cover.
- Most people are not familiar with cross sections of anatomy, so choose uncluttered pictures that show clearly what you want to explain.
- Make sure the charts and the details you point out are clearly visible to everyone in the room.
- Help people orientate themselves by identifying landmarks that you have already talked about. 'Here is the pubic bone and here's the tail-bone.'
- Where possible, use life-size diagrams and hold them against your body in the correct position so they can see where the 'part' fits into the 'whole'.
- When using charts to show the progress of the baby during labour, hold them upright rather than horizontally. This demonstrates the benefits of being upright and mobile during labour.

Slides

There are dozens of commercially produced sets on offer which you can tailor to meet your own needs by picking the images you want and leaving out those you don't. Timing is in your control, so you can stop and talk over one slide, then go quickly through less interesting ones. However, slides of labour lose the dynamic, changing, exciting pace of birth itself and can give a distorted view. Leaving a very large image of a head crowning on for more than a few seconds makes the woman look stuck and desperate.

Like many audio-visual aids, slides date very quickly and have the disadvantage of turning your group into an audience. You will find it hard to judge reactions when people sit in the dark, facing away from you. Slides also require energy and organization to get the equipment ready. Unless you can find a set that really adds to what you can offer with your own actions, photos and demonstrations, you will need to consider carefully whether slides are worth the effort.

Videos

When we ask a group of antenatal teachers to brainstorm what visual aids they might use, videos usually head the list. There are several reasons for this, only some of which are geared to more effective classes:

- Videos give the teacher a rest. This can be a valuable use of time in a busy, stressful day. Twenty minutes spent catching your breath while they watch a video can mean you are truly available for the rest of the session.
- Videos bring variety and another version of reality into the group. Teachers who find acting out contractions or pretending to be desperate with a crying baby difficult will be tempted to use a video rather than developing their own ability to mimic it.
- Videos offer another point of view. Lots of them include several parents sharing views and telling their own stories.

Many parents expect to see a video of a birth and feel cheated without one. There may be a place for a short (20 minutes or so), up-to-date video of a birth as long as it includes a commentary you feel is suitable and it has been shot from the parents' point of view rather than the midwife's. A video that focuses on a larger-than-life, bulging perineum can upset some people. The mother will certainly not have this view of her own labour and a father who is supporting his partner is unlikely to either.

Another useful kind of video lasts only a few minutes and triggers activity. If a video leaves a group gingered up to discuss an issue or try out some positions, it is useful.

However, many parents have already seen videos or TV programmes on birth and are keen for something else. They often show this by talking through the video. A group that reacts in this way is telling you they recognize the unique opportunity that being in an antenatal class offers them and they are reluctant to spend it as a passive audience. The disadvantage of videos for the teacher include expense, problems with equipment, compensating for out-of-date or inappropriate information, and the annoyance of watching the same thing, again and again. These may well outweigh the advantages. You will need to do that particular equation for yourself.

In conclusion

Choosing and using visual aids effectively takes thought, planning and practice. We have found that the cheapest, most available, flexible and most effective visual aid is ourselves. It's well worth setting aside your inhibitions and taking the risk of showing parents to the best of your ability, what labour or feeding or caring for a new baby *really* is like.

15

Team-teaching

It is very common for two or more people to be involved in running an antenatal course. Sometimes, responsibility for the class passes from one teacher to another with little or no chance for them to meet. When a course is organized like this, the hope is that parents will build the separate bits into a coherent whole rather like patches making up a quilt.

There are real drawbacks to this 'patchwork' approach to antenatal teaching. Parents can miss out on the benefits of group work because it is difficult if not impossible to create or maintain a group if the leadership changes frequently. Without group experiences, parents never get to know each other, so the social benefits disappear. People may never get to know the teacher well enough to feel able to ask difficult questions or bring up sensitive issues. Drop-out is likely to be high and satisfaction low.

This way of running classes also creates problems for the teacher. If she is given responsibility for running only a small portion of the course and responsibility for only certain topics, skills or ideas, then her ability to react to what is happening in the class is very limited. She may not have the necessary skills to deal with a topic that is brought up by the class or she may be limited in her ability to change the pace and type of activity in response to unexpected changes of mood or need. With no notion of how her teaching fits in to the whole, it can become mechanical or ritualized. She may also lose out on feedback on her portion of the course as a whole.

One way around these problems is to assign one teacher for the whole course. That's what is presumed in most of the other chapters in this book. This chapter looks at another solution to the difficulties that can arise when two or more people teach a course. We call it team-teaching, and it only happens when everyone who runs the course thinks together, plans together and reviews together. They may or may not actually teach together (few managers feel able to allocate two people to a session, given present staffing levels), but a team can still be a reality if the members have an equal commitment to making the course work, share equal responsibility for what happens, and put themselves across to the parents as a unit.

Benefits of team-teaching

Many teachers will prefer to work alone. But if you do share the task of running a course, then the benefits of teamwork amply repay the time and effort needed to operate in this way. In a team, there is someone to think and plan with; someone to bounce ideas off; to learn from; to give constructive feedback; to listen when the going gets tough; and someone to have fun with! It eases the isolation many teachers feel. The product, whether it be a book like this one or an antenatal course, is likely to be improved as a result of having input from two heads rather than one. Your group, too, will benefit from having two (or more) teachers because they offer different teaching styles and more models to copy so parents are more likely to find one that's right for them (see Fig. 14.6 on page 142).

Steps to good teamwork

The steps listed below will only work when all participants offer their honesty and trust. This may be a slow process, so make sure you and your partner give each other the time you need.

- Invite your partner to spend some time with you, thinking about the way you work or could work together.
- Arrange a time and place where you can be together without interruption. It may help to agree on confidentiality and it is important that you are careful to take equal time to talk and listen.
- Depending on how well you know each other, find out a bit about each other, possibly including your life outside work.
- Spend some time listening to each other's aims and approach to leading antenatal classes.
- Listen carefully and respectfully to your differences. They could enrich rather than cause problems. If necessary talk them through, now or later, and seek compromise and balance.
- Take turns to talk about what you enjoy doing. What you are good at. Then, what you find hard or dislike doing.

- Talk about what you like (or think you will like) about working together. Then, about what might be hard or could be improved.
- Identify ways in which you could enhance each other's skills and abilities.
- End by each of you saying what you have liked or found helpful about looking at the way you work together and plan ahead for regular reviews.

At follow-up meetings, build in time to review what has gone well since you last met and identify areas that need attention. Then work together, perhaps planning a course using small cards as we described in Chapter 5. You might think through a problem, possibly using a large sheet of paper to catch and record each other's thoughts, or review your teaching using the format suggested in Chapter 21. You could also discuss some of the issues we have raised in this chapter or deal with those that have come up as a result of your work together.

Some team-teaching issues

Institutional inhibitions

If you want to try team-teaching, things may hold you back. It might be the management who have always run classes one way and don't wish to change. Or the person organizing timetables who wants to cover sickness or holidays. Often, co-operation is hampered when health professionals guard certain skills or knowledge as belonging to themselves alone. Chapter 20 on initiating change, may help you get started at tackling these blocks.

Your own feelings and fears

The good news is, these are the obstacles you are most able to do something about as we have certainly found in our years of working together. We may feel possessive and not want to share the work. We may feel threatened by each other's ideas and skills or unwilling to share our own, eirher because we fear they are not good enough, or because someone else might steal them! Or we may feel superior or irritated by some of the things our partner does or does not do. But we keep trying and keep talking together about the things that might get in our way.

Getting started as a team

Once you are working as a team, how will you divide up the teaching and build and maintain the group together? Will you start the first class jointly? This has many advantages. You both participate in the initial introductions and if you are setting ground rules or finding out what the participants want, you are both part of the process. People get to know you both at the same time and are more likely to view you as a team.

Changing teachers

If you do not start the group jointly, how will you prepare the class for a change of leadership? It is very hard, particularly as the teacher, to come into a group that has already been working together and which knows what to expect of the teacher. Group members may feel apprehensive or resentful of having to make another adjustment. The new teacher may also feel anxious about meeting people who already know each other and who may compare her to her colleague.

The way you prepare the class for a change of teacher is important. The participants need to know from the outset that the teaching will be shared. The words you use to tell them are only a small part of the message you convey. If you simply inform them that someone else will lead the next session, they may feel let down or even abandoned. This makes a difficult task even harder for the second teacher. If, on the other hand you set the scene for co-teaching right from the start of the course and speak of your colleague with warmth, as you would speak of one friend to another friend, the class will be more receptive. If, for some reason, you do not warm to your co-teacher, at least speak of her with respect.

Working flexibly

How are you going to decide who does what? You don't have to stick to rigid roles, professional boundaries or old ways of working. Everyone can learn to lead effective relaxation sessions, just as all teachers can develop the skills needed to start and maintain good group discussion. You'll find suggestions for both elsewhere in this book. Teamwork may be an opportunity for both teachers to develop new skills, with the unusual advantage of having each other to learn from.

As your own repertoire grows, you can vary activities according to the immediate needs and mood of the group rather than the agreed schedule or the preconceived domains of any one person. For example, if the plan was to cover the early postnatal experience but the group is sluggish and unresponsive, you might decide to practise second stage positions instead. Another day, in a discussion on obstetric interventions you could get the message that what they really want to discuss is last night's television programme on immunization. You can switch *if* you have already agreed this style of leading with your colleagues and have organized a form of record-keeping that allows spontaneous changes of plans without losing the thread of the course (see page 38 for one way of doing this).

Exchanging information

Telling each other what happened and what you have learned about the individuals attending the course is vital, but this has to be balanced with confidentiality, especially if you have agreed this in the group's ground rules.

Health professionals are used to exchanging confidential information about patients as part of the care they offer. But should this automatically extend to information given in an antenatal discussion group or to an individual teacher?

In conclusion

Much of this chapter refers to two co-teachers but could apply equally well to teams with more members. The larger the group, the more time and discussion will be needed before everyone feels involved, included and respected. However many are on your team, when you team-teach, you model co-operation and compromise, tolerance and communication. This is of direct relevance to the parents you teach. Those who are in long-term relationships are preparing to take on their own joint venture – looking after a baby. When they are parents, they will need to find out about each other's views, beliefs and opinions about child rearing and to identify their own and their partner's strengths and weaknesses. They will have to accept that there is more than one way of doing most things and work for compromise. Your demonstration of flexibility and respect for each other's skills and points of view will be more effective than anything you could tell them about how they themselves might become a team.

Further reading

The International Standard Book Number (ISBN) is given where possible and should be quoted when ordering the book from your bookseller.

General books on antenatal teaching

Billingham, Kate (1990) *Learning Together – a health resource pack for working with groups,* available from Kate Billingham, Nottingham Community Unit, Memorial House, Standard Hill, Nottingham NG1 6FX [Collected ideas of someone who ran community-based classes. Full of suggestions for involving the group.]

Cronk, Mary and Flint, Caroline (1989) *Community Midwifery – A Practical Guide,* Heinemann Medical Books, London (ISBN 0-433-00017-1) [Contains a useful chapter on antenatal classes.]

Kitzinger, Sheila (1977) *Education and Counselling for Childbirth,* Baillière Tindall, London (ISBN 0-7020-0642-4) [Strong on the sensitive listening and open-minded acceptance teachers need.]

Murphy-Black, Tricia and Faulkner, Ann (1988) *Antenatal Skills – A Manual of Guidelines,* John Wiley and Sons, Chichester (ISBN 0-471-91138-0) [Aimed at tutors and parentcraft co-ordinators who want to help others learn to run classes well.]

Noble, Elizabeth (1983) *Childbirth with Insight,* Houghton Mifflin, Boston, USA (ISBN 0-395-33962-6) [How one experienced teacher wishes antenatal classes were run. Available from the National Childbirth Trust – see Appendix I.]

PIPSI (1990) *Progressive and Innovative Parentcraft Teachers Support and Interest Group – activity pack,* available from PIPSI – see Appendix I

Robertson, Andrea (1988) *Teaching Active Birth – A Handbook for Childbirth Educators and Midwives,* ACE Graphics (ISBN 0-958801-5-17), available from Midwives' Information and Resources Service – see Appendix I

Wilson, Patricia (1989) *Antenatal Teaching,* Faber, London (ISBN 0-571-14113-7)

Books with suggestions for physical skills

Dale, Barbara and Roeber, Johanna (1991) *Exercises for Childbirth,* Frances Lincoln, London (ISBN 0-7112-0678-3) [Good, clear photographs and easy-to-follow directions. Very useful.]

Gawain, Shakti (1985) *Creative Visualisation,* Bantam New Age Books, New York (ISBN 0-553-24147-8)

Kitzinger, Sheila (1987) *The Experience of Childbirth,* Penguin, Harmondsworth (ISBN 0-14-02. 0900X) [One of the classics. Good instructions on touch relaxation.]

Kravette, Steve (1979) *Complete Relaxation,* Para Research (ISBN 0-91-491-814-1) [Full of ideas to stimulate imaginative teaching and use of relaxation.]

Leboyer, Frederic (1985) *The Art of Breathing,* Element Books, Shaftesbury (ISBN 0-906540-82-8)

Madders, Jane (1987) *Relax and Be Happy,* Unwin, London (ISBN 0-04-649043-4) [Aimed primarily at teaching children to relax. Full of short, fun techniques and some good scripts for longer work.]

Mitchell, Laura (1988) *Simple Relaxation,* Murray, London (ISBN 0-7195-4388-6)

O'Brien, Paddy (1988) *Birth and Our Bodies,* Pandora, London (ISBN 086-358-0475) [Includes exercises and yoga for pregnancy and birth, plus sections on relaxation.]

Whitford, Barbara and Polden, Margie (1988) *Postnatal Exercises,* Century Hutchinson (ISBN 0-7126-2464-3)

Aids to help you teach breastfeeding

Breastfeeding workshops devised by Lea Jamieson. A 'hands off' approach to enable midwives to assist mothers to start and maintain breastfeeding. For information contact Garden Flat 5, Clifton Avenue, London W12 9DR. Tel: 081-743-4417.

Minchin, Maureen (1985) *Breastfeeding Matters,* Alma Publications, available from the National Childbirth Trust – see Appendix I (ISBN 0-86861-810)

Renfrew, Mary, Fisher, Chloe and Arms, Suzanne (1990) *Best feeding – Getting Breastfeeding Right For You,* Celestial Arts, available from the National Childbirth Trust or the Midwives' Information and Resource Service – see Appendix I

Royal College of Midwives (1991) *Successful Breastfeeding – A Practical Guide for Midwives and Others Supporting Breastfeeding Mothers* (2nd edn), Churchill Livingstone, Edinburgh

Books on groupwork and active learning

Henderson, Penny (1985) *Promoting Active Learning,* National Extension College – see Appendix I (ISBN 1-85356-029-4)

Houston, Gaie (1984) *The Red Book of Groups,* The Rochester Foundation, 8 Rochester Terrace, London NW1 [A practical book for those wanting to develop their skills.]

Kindred, Michael (1985) *Once Upon a Group,* available from the author at 20 Dover Street, Southwell, Notts NG25 0EZ (£3 + 0.40p for postage) [An entertaining book which takes the mystery out of how groups behave and how to lead them.]

Other useful books

Bond, Meg (1987) *Stress and Self-Awareness – A Guide for Nurses*, Heinemann, London (ISBN 0-433-03490-4) [A down-to-earth approach for all those wishing to look after themselves well.]

Welford, Heather (1987) *Illustrated Dictionary of Pregnancy and Birth*, Unwin, London (ISBN 0-04-612047-5) [Full of user-friendly ways of describing procedures and happenings.]

Visual aids

See Appendix II for sources of visual aids.

Part III

Fine-tuning your antenatal course

16

Preparing for parenthood

Labour, crucial though it is in a woman's life, seldom lasts longer than 24 hours. Parenthood lasts years – decades! Being a parent is the only job that people are expected to do, often in isolation, without help or support, for 24 hours a day, 7 days a week, 52 weeks a year. Most of us start out with virtually no preparation save our own experience of being parented. Many hold a new baby for the first time when their own is placed in their arms. The commonest cry heard at postnatal reunions is, 'Why didn't somebody *tell* me it would be like this?'.

These factors make the case for more preparation for parenthood seem overwhelming, but is the antenatal class the right place? When a woman is pregnant, especially the first time, labour and birth loom very large. They seem to form an almost tangible barrier between her current life and the one to come. Antenatal teachers, too, often say they concentrate on pregnancy and labour because it is so hard to encourage expectant parents to see 'over the wall' to parenthood.

But this understandably narrow focus has several negative aspects. First, it may perpetuate the myth that birth is the end of the story. It is not unusual for women to sigh, 'Thank God it is all over', one minute after their babies are born. In fact, 'it' is just beginning. Second, looking just towards birth encourages the strange notion that people only become parents once the baby is born. Ask a pregnant woman, 'Who is looking after this baby?' and a surprising number answer with the name of their consultant obstetrician. Yet it is their body that nurtures and protects their baby and they have already made dozens – hundreds – of decisions themselves on the baby's behalf. Finally, concentrating only on life before birth because parents find it hard to look at life after birth fails to encourage everyone – parents and antenatal teachers – to think creatively about the major changes that the arrival of a new baby will bring.

Thinking beyond birth

Labour and birth may seem like a barrier beyond which expectant parents cannot see clearly. They are only able to 'jump' (in their imagination) high enough for a brief look over. Your job is to make those glimpses as vivid as possible, offering a realistic picture of what lies ahead. One good way is to weave in references to the baby and to life after birth throughout the course. The key step is to focus on the babies in the room as sensitive, feeling individuals. You can do this by one of the means described below.

Acknowledging their presence

When someone is taking a count for coffee, ask, 'How many people are there in this room?'

When you demonstrate a new position for labour and the manoeuvre jostles the baby, apologize directly. 'Sorry, little one. You were comfortable before we started all this, eh?'

Talk about 'your baby' rather than 'your bump'.

Say, 'Your baby's grown this week' instead of, 'Aren't you big!'.

When a woman announces, 'I'm engaged!', remind her gently who *really* is.

Encouraging parents to identify their baby's individual quirks

Each baby has his or her own patterns of activity and rest. Some are prone to hiccups. Some seem to quieten when the father puts his hand on the mother's tummy. A few object when a woman sits for too long. Start a class with a round asking, 'How has your baby been this week?' or 'What does he like?', 'What does she dislike?'.

Offering basic information

The babies are already able to suck, swallow, hear and dimly to perceive light. At birth, they will recognize the voices of their parents and may be soothed by music that they heard before they were born. Chapter 12 suggests ways to combine giving this kind of information with relaxation.

Providing powerful images

No babies are 'it', so use 'he' or 'she' when talking about them, alternating the sex frequently. Handle the doll often and with respect, as gently as you would a real baby (see Chapter 14). Invite back a couple or a mother with a baby under six weeks old. Over that age and parents can't relate the baby they see with the one inside. You will need to take care when choosing whom to ask back. Page 169 offers more suggestions about inviting in parents.

Linking every topic to the baby

What might contractions be like for the baby? What might it be like for the baby to emerge into the world? What welcome would he or she appreciate? What are the effects of various procedures on the baby? What is it like for the baby to be monitored? What are the effects on the baby of pethidine? An epidural? Entonox?

Drawing analogies between current experiences and parenthood

The unpredictable and inevitable nature of labour is like the erratic and continuous needs of a new baby. The disturbed sleep of late pregnancy mirrors broken nights after the birth. Babies literally come between a couple who want to hug in pregnancy and are just as intrusive once born. One mother said, 'Two of my three children were very active before they were born and they are the ones who can't sit still!'

Making time to plan for parenthood

If you decide to focus specifically on life after birth, one place to start is with teaching practical skills like comforting a crying baby or baby massage. Choose skills that are unlikely to be taught in hospital or which become so much more relevant once a baby is born (like bathing). Also avoid skills that nearly everyone picks up for themselves such as nappy changing.

Many teachers set aside one or two classes towards the end of a course for demonstration, practice and discussion of postnatal issues. Others intersperse postnatal topics with those concentrating on pregnancy or labour. The latter plan is often a happy combination because everyday, useful topics help lift the mood should the discussion turn sombre. Concrete issues like what to buy for a baby offer a welcome contrast to ones where women try to imagine what labour is like or what will help them cope.

Another way to look ahead is to encourage expectant parents to share their ideas about parenthood. This is usually more successful towards the end of a course when the imminence of birth makes these ideas more real. Think carefully about the question(s) you ask to get a discussion going. Hypothetical ones are usually met with blank looks e.g. 'How do you think this baby will change your life?'. Try something more concrete like: 'What have you seen your friends who already have children doing/not doing that made you think, "I'll never do that . . ."?' Or 'In what ways will you raise your baby differently from the ways your parents brought you up, and in what ways will you follow your own parents' example?'

Talking and listening to others helps expectant parents see how many different ways there are to care for babies. As different ideas emerge, you need to help the group listen respectfully to whoever offers them. Almost always, ideas about parenthood are neither right nor wrong, better nor worse – just different. If you hear ideas that make you uneasy, wait to see if the group will counter them with other thoughts before trying yourself to reshape what was said (see Chapter 7 for gentle ways of doing this).

Another way to combine antenatal and postnatal issues is to point out how the skills you teach for pregnancy and birth can be useful once the baby is born. 'Relaxation makes a tense parent more able to comfort a distressed baby'; 'Many babies love to be massaged'; 'Communication skills learned for labour will come in handy with GPs and Health Visitors, too.'

Finally, there is a whole host of activities designed to raise awareness of the changes the new baby will make to everyday life, to relationships and to daily routines. Chapter 10 suggests several as do the books listed at the end of Parts II and III. There are all kinds of ways to encourage parents to start thinking for themselves about meeting the new challenges that lie ahead. Of course, it is unrealistic to think that a six- or eight-week course is adequate preparation for parenthood, but it can be a start.

17

Working with fathers

Twenty-five years ago, a man who wanted to be present at the birth of his child or who pushed a pram in the street was thought to be rather odd. Now, a man who does *not* want to do these things is quite likely to receive pressure and teasing, often from other men. This is, of course, a generalization and attitudes vary a great deal depending on class, cultural group or geographical area. Nevertheless, it is true for a significant proportion of expectant and new fathers.

Over the same period of time, the place of men in antenatal classes has evolved too, although here the changes have usually been less radical than in the wider world. In the beginning, fathers were not involved at all. Then fathers' evenings were included. Later, courses for couples were introduced. When these changes were made without careful inclusion of the father's perspective, men often felt patronized or found themselves being cast purely in the role of supporter with their own needs ignored.

This chapter looks at the importance of incorporating the father's needs and perspectives throughout the course, whether or not men are actually physically present the whole time. The chapter also examines the pressures on men during pregnancy, including those caused by antenatal classes. It then suggests ways of working with expectant fathers (as well as their pregnant partners), so that men feel included and cared for in your class. Some of the suggestions will need modifying should you decide to run a course which is mostly for women with one or two sessions where fathers are included.

Your attitudes on working with men

The whole question of men in antenatal classes can stir strong feelings. Just as we can nearly always get parents talking with the statement, 'A woman's place is in the home', so suggesting to a group of teachers that a man's place is or isn't in their class is bound to generate comment. How do you feel about men being in your class?

For some antenatal teachers, having men in the class can be problematic. They may not be sure why men come and do not like the effect men's presence can have on the group. Some teachers feel that, in a mixed group, men often inhibit women from talking freely, or distract the group with anything from too many jokes to outright hostility. Some teachers, when pressed, admit they feel anxious about teaching men because they find it hard to believe that men will take them seriously.

Other teachers feel more positive about working with men. They say that men widen the scope of classes and that having them there simply reflects the reality of two-parent families. Having both men and women in the group greatly increases the over-all richness and variety that make a group work well.

It may take some time to work out your own feelings about mixed-sex classes. Any planning for men must start with your own attitudes since these will set the tone of your classes far more than the teaching techniques or particular exercises you select. Your own attitudes may also tip the balance for or against inviting men into your class (although, of course, some teachers have the decision made for them). Even if you are a reluctant co-educationalist, you will work better with men if you can understand what brings them to classes and accept that they, like the women they accompany, have real needs. By thinking about the men, you will actually benefit the women who are with them because running *good* classes for men allows the women to relax and pay attention to their own needs rather than worry if their partners are bored, angry or alienated.

Men expecting babies

Men, too, are prospective parents. They face change and challenge. Many will have high expectations of themselves. Their partners' expectations for them may be higher still. 'New man' is probably two-thirds media creation and one-third middle class myth but, for all the hype, his influence is pretty powerful. Today's man is expected to be gentle, sensitive and aware both during labour and as a father. In large sections of the community, unless men do their share of nappy changing and baby comforting they are in danger of being called selfish and unsupportive.

So much for the expectations. How are men supposed to learn to do these things? By and large, their fathers didn't behave like this, so their own childhood memories offer few clues. Even if there were lots of 'new men' around, they wouldn't be much help to the novice father because men rarely talk about domestic issues, and even more rarely say how they feel about them. The end result is that men arrive in class having had few if any opportunities to explore their own hopes and fears or to learn practical skills from each other. They may also have very mixed feelings about going to antenatal classes at all.

For many men, classes are one of the many hurdles they encounter during pregnancy. 'It was', said one man, 'like entering a women's Masonic lodge.' Many come reluctantly, especially the first time. Some find the whole idea acutely embarrassing; others are genuinely worried about what might be expected of them.

Labour, too, can pull men in different directions. Many will be entranced by the technology of birth. Some may be terrified and squeamish. More than a few harbour deep fears of death, mutilation and humiliation. Some will already have children from previous relationships and one or two, perhaps unbeknown to their current partners, may be reminded of babies they fathered that were aborted. In fact, their thoughts and feelings will be as vivid and varied as those of the women they accompany.

Finding out what men think and need

In order to tailor your course to meet men's needs, you must know what these needs are. People who lead antenatal classes tend to be more aware of the practical and emotional needs of pregnant women than of expectant fathers. If that's true of you, you should take any opportunity you can to invite men to talk about their needs and feelings and then listen really well.

Ask male friends, relatives, colleagues or men who come to your classes. Compare the differences between men who have become fathers recently with those of many years ago. You may learn more if you listen to a man on his own, because many men hold back on the issues that really bother them to protect their partners.

There is a whole range of questions you could ask to give you the insights you need to work well with expectant fathers:

> How did you feel during your partner's pregnancy? What changes did you notice in yourself? Who or what helped you if you needed it?
>
> What was it like for you coming to classes? What was good? What was hard? What else would have been useful?
>
> What was it like for you being at the labour and at your baby's birth? Where could you get support if you needed it?
>
> What was it like leaving your partner and your baby in hospital after the birth? What made it easier/harder?
>
> In what ways did your father look after you when you were very little? Was he there for your birth? What feelings do you bring to this experience from your childhood?

In time, you will hear a wide range of experiences and begin to recognize common themes and topics. Being in touch with men will help you gauge whether or not your classes are about right for the fathers in your group and will tell you how to make changes appropriate to their needs.

Welcoming and involving fathers

Men can't just be tacked on to a woman's course – they have to be included all along the way, from planning and publicity to the actual work you do together in the class. If you plan a course for both men and women, make sure the men know about it in advance, too. Whether you invite men to a couples' course or to a fathers' evening(s) within a women's course, reflect your welcome in any written material you use and in the verbal information you give to the women. If you invite the class to set the agenda for the course, or for the father's evening, it is important to ensure that the issues raised by the men are covered.

Look at every topic and activity from the father's point of view both as a support for his partner and as a person in his own right. For example, for a fathers' evening, you could ask yourself:

> What will he see, hear or touch? What feelings will the experience trigger in him? What information will he need to make sense of what is happening?
>
> What could he do to support his partner? What can he do to take care of his own needs and feelings?

You might find standing in a man's shoes surprisingly hard. Let us consider how this might be done by focusing on a sample topic. How could you talk with a mixed group about episiotomy? There are certain things both men and women need to know such as when, how and why it is done. Women particularly need to know other things – what the snip feels like, that local anaesthesia sometimes stings, how looking with a mirror afterwards will help them get a true picture of the scar size, or the various ways in which they can speed healing. Men, on the other hand, are often glad to know that the snip itself is audible and to be offered ways of coping: 'Hum quietly when the midwife picks up the scissors.' They may welcome suggestions on more comfortable love-making afterwards: 'Keep pressure off the back of the vagina. . .'. Or you might suggest ways to help a woman as she is being stitched. When you cover a topic in this way, some of the class is 'eavesdropping', so you need to switch from one to the other frequently, clearly signalling whom you are addressing.

As well as topics common to both men and women, think about the things that only fathers may experience. For example:

- arranging to leave work at a moment's notice when labour starts;
- being left abruptly outside the theatre during an emergency caesarian;
- being separated from his partner and baby when he leaves the hospital after the birth;
- juggling the demands of a job, visiting hospital, keeping home in some semblance of order and fielding calls from relatives;
- negotiating paternity leave or days off work to be with his partner and baby when they come home from hospital.

One activity that men seem particularly grateful to discuss is what we call 'How to Catch a Baby in the Kitchen'. This has the double utility of easing their anxiety and convincing them that the classes are just as much for their benefit as for their partner's. If you describe an emergency delivery, make it as realistic as possible: 'Here, hold your hand over my fist. I'll be the baby's head and you make sure it doesn't come too fast. . . . Gently, gently.' Obviously, you must offer plenty of reassurance that this is very, very rare and that delivering a baby if you are not trained to do so is not only foolish and dangerous, it is punishable by law if there is time to get help. You may find this a useful activity to do with the men if you split the class into different-sex groups in an early session of the course.

Language

Every word you use in a mixed group must apply to him too. Instead of 'your uterus' try 'the uterus'. Instead of 'when you have a contraction' you could say 'when the next contraction comes . . .'. If you are speaking only to the women, preface your comment with something that denotes this, like: 'Now you women, when you do X . . .'. If there are only one or two men in the group, you will need to preface comments directed at the women less often, but it will still be necessary regularly to show that you are aware of the men in the room.

You may also need to consider the generic term you use for people in the room who are not pregnant. Most teachers have abandoned 'husbands' long ago, but what word(s) will replace it? Partners? Dads? Fellahs? You men? In this whole section, we have presumed that a couple is heterosexual. How will you address a group where this isn't so? Perhaps you have a lesbian couple or a woman and her friend or mother. All these variations will demand a change in the words you use.

It can be difficult to use gender-appropriate language consistently. Many of us have developed patterns of speech directed primarily towards women and it will take time and effort to change. One way to start is to review what you say, topic by topic, considering the phrases you usually use. If you work with someone, you might come to an agreement whereby both of you keep an ear open for phrases that exclude the fathers. Or ask the group to help you. (See Chapter 8 for a more general discussion on the use of language.)

Practical work

Always involve men in practice sessions when teaching physical skills. Some may be very reluctant to take part, but with gentle encouragement most can be persuaded that joining in will be less awkward than sitting as a spectator. Invite them to try out relaxation and breathing for themselves. Offer time for men to receive massage as well as to give it. Encourage them to help their partners find comfortable positions and to explore ways of supporting their partners both physically and emotionally.

In all these activities, make sure that men look after themselves. Watch posture and positioning, so they avoid straining their backs when they support or massage their partners. Acknowledge how tiring it can be helping a woman in labour. Look at ways to ease the harder bits and identify the things men can do to conserve their energy. These will include eating regularly and taking time for a stretch and perhaps a breath of fresh air.

Peer support

Antenatal classes can offer men a unique opportunity to be with other men in the same situation. You can maximize the benefits of this by providing opportunities for men to talk together. You might, for

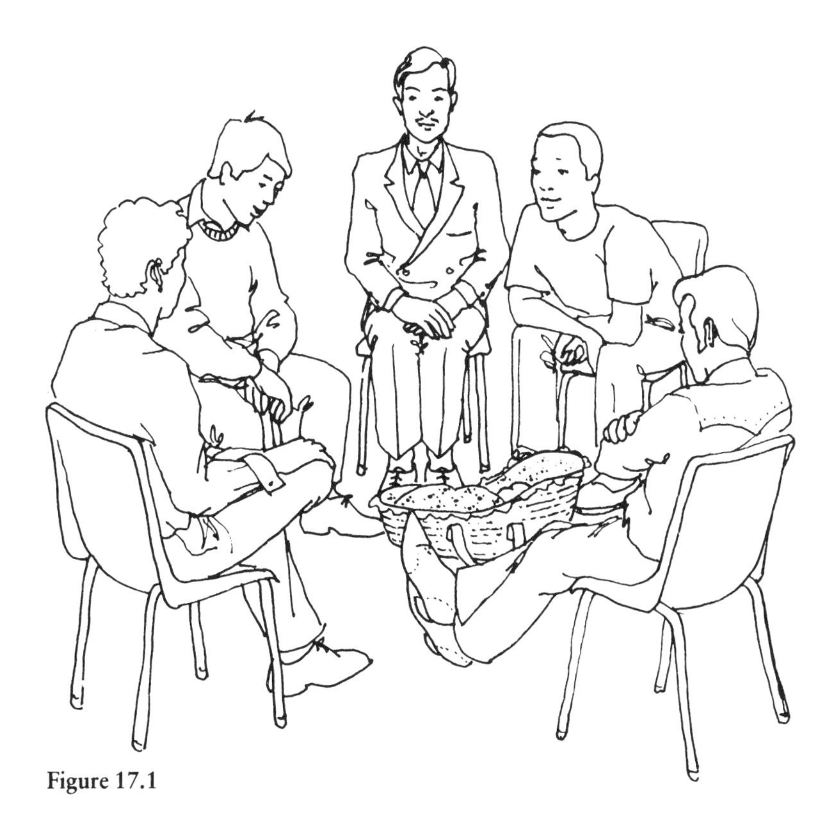

Figure 17.1

example, divide the class into single-sex groups, then invite each to discuss a topic from their own perspective. Questions might include:

> What excites you about the prospect of labour? What worries you?
>
> What are the things you are most looking forward to about becoming a father/mother? What are the things you are least looking forward to?
>
> What help and support would you like from your partner in the first few days after your baby is born?

Small group discussions don't always need to be shared with the larger group. Sometimes, simply giving people time and safety in which to talk and listen is enough. Not reporting back often spurs couples into talking together after the class. If you don't plan to have a large-group discussion, make this known when you set up the groups. Remind people that anything that is said in their group must remain confidential or be shared in a way that respects others' anonymity.

At other times, you *will* want subgroups to report back and, here again, they need to know both if and how it is to be done before they begin. One way to do this that preserves confidentiality is to ask groups to summarize their discussions on a chart. The charts can then be displayed and discussed in a way which still maintains confidentiality for individuals. This often triggers an interesting exchange about the different and similar perspectives of men and women.

Offering positive images

Because men have few models and the images of new fathers reflected by the media are often idealized or mocking, you can help them by offering realistic and practical insights into fatherhood. One way of doing this is to start a discussion on what men have heard from their male friends and relatives about being at the birth and becoming a father.

Another way is to invite a new father to talk about his experience of labour, birth and the early days of parenting. You can set this up as an informal discussion group or guide the conversation by asking the father questions that will encourage him to discuss certain issues. Include questions that invite him to talk about his reactions and feelings as well as about factual events.

Think carefully when deciding who to invite. The ideal candidate is neither long-winded nor dogmatic. Do you want somebody whose partner had an easy, straightforward labour, someone with a long and difficult story to tell, or doesn't it matter? Will he come alone or bring his baby? Will his partner come and, if so, what will her role be? Will she listen while he talks about his experience or will you give her time as well?

You also convey images through some of the visual aids you use. Many visual aids marginalize the father, focusing instead on the woman and midwife. This is especially true of slides and videos which should ideally depict an involved and active man. If your visual aids only show an anxious-looking father, sitting awkwardly in the corner, draw the group's attention to this and encourage a discussion about what that man might be feeling. Ask them to consider how he could move from bystander to active participant.

In conclusion

Antenatal classes can serve a unique function for men who may have no other forum in which to think about their own feelings or talk with other men in the same situation. By focusing on men's needs and perspectives *as people in their own right*, not just in their role as supporters or companions, you can offer women new insights about their partners, and men a valuable opportunity to prepare for the enormous changes and demands that fatherhood brings.

18

Groups with shared needs

Some expectant parents will have particular needs when it comes to antenatal preparation. In this chapter, we explore some of the issues and look at how some of these needs might be met.

Parents expecting second and subsequent babies

You can address the needs and concerns of people having second or subsequent babies in two ways. You can either make time within a class designed primarily for first-time parents, or design and run a course just for them.

Integrated classes

There are many good reasons – not least of which might be low numbers or limited resources – for running one programme and inviting everyone regardless of parity. An integrated class offers several benefits to experienced parents. They can tell their stories and understand more fully what happened last time. They can also update their information and renew contacts with other pregnant women, something that is particularly important if there has been a wide gap between children. Parents' confidence often increases as they compare their current state of mind with the uncertainty of first-time parents. And people who didn't go to classes for their first baby will learn a great deal from everything you offer the class.

However, experienced parents probably give more than they receive in a mixed class. Thanks to their broader vision and experience, the group is richer and you as teacher can draw on their insights to illustrate information, trigger discussion and make the birth process vivid. As recompense, they deserve special effort from you. For example, when addressing the whole group, you need to make sure the language you use and the examples you cite are appropriate to everyone, not just those expecting a first baby (see Chapter 8).

Other ways to make space for experienced parents include forming a subgroup for some discussions, perhaps to address issues like those described in the next section, while first-timers focus on other things. Often, experienced parents like practising physical skills together because they can be less inhibited and are more able to grasp their purpose. You could even include one session in a mixed course specifically for experienced parents.

Separate classes

Another way to meet the needs of experienced parents is to offer them a course of their own to deal primarily with their concerns. To plan such a course, you can use the same process we described in Chapter 5. How many classes will you run and who will be invited? Will you run an open or closed group and what topics will you include? If you use the card method described in Chapter 5, you need different topics so start by making a new list of the information, physical skills and attitudes and feelings you think could be usefully explored with experienced parents. However, because experienced parents are more likely to know what they need, be prepared to be very flexible and responsive to what they want.

Some of their needs are fairly easy to predict. They need to talk about their last labour(s) so they can feel free to experience the one to come. Only a lucky few will have done this already, leaving the rest full of undigested birth stories just waiting to be told. This 'debriefing' is more effective if it is done in a systematic way. Each person is offered the chance to be heard, to make more sense of what happened and to share feelings and experiences. Now and again, you will encounter someone whose experiences were so traumatic that she needs more time or more skill than can be offered in class. Counselling or other specialized help may be called for.

There are several ways you can help group members tell their stories. They can write down what happened, although the less literary or those whose first language is not English may find this difficult. In a small group, of not more than six, you might set up a round where each person has a predetermined amount of time to speak while the others just listen. Even five minutes of uninterrupted attention, where no one advises, judges or side-tracks with her own history, can be a powerful experience. You could find that most people want more than this amount of time. If so, encourage the group to make this decision and make sure the additional time is shared equally.

In a large group, break them into twos or threes, making sure that the listeners know that they must not interrupt and that everyone deserves equal time. This encourages the more silent to speak, ensures that people unused to listening do not have too many stories to take in, and allows each speaker a reasonable amount of time.

Even after this kind of 'debriefing', a few people will return to their experiences again and again. They may need more listening, either within the group or elsewhere. If the group has an agreement about equal time (see Chapter 6), referring to it may help them hold back from monopolizing the group.

Telling the story is the first step towards making sense of what happened. To help the process further, people could consider open questions such as: 'What is the most important thing you learned from the experience?' 'How did it change you?' 'What was the most helpful person/action?' And 'How does it affect your hopes and fears for *this* pregnancy?' '*This* labour?' '*This* baby?' In time, they may feel sufficiently free of the last experience to begin to look towards the next.

As well as looking backwards, most parents will want to plan ahead. Experienced parents often say that the main benefit of going to classes is having time away from their busy lives to acknowledge *this* baby and *this* impending birth. They also have a much clearer picture of what they want and what they can expect of themselves and others. Practical skills are no longer strange rituals, but linked to known feelings and imaginable happenings. And many are experienced consumers, able to judge what they need to know and from whom (and that includes you).

Experienced parents are often also keen to look beyond birth and they want to think about how *this* baby will fit into the family. Most of the practical babycare issues are already solved but parents may, for example, be concerned about who will look after the first child so that the father can be with the mother during labour. How will the fathers cope with both caring for the first child and spending time with his partner and new baby? How will grandparents, work mates or friends react?

Above all, many parents are anxious about how they will make space in their lives and their hearts for another child when the first seems so all-absorbing. They may be keen to discuss normal reactions to a new baby, sibling rivalry and possible ways to ease the transition from only child to big brother or sister. Some of the active learning exercises described in Chapter 10 work particularly well with experienced parents on just such matters.

Parents with multiple families

One issue that may arise in any antenatal group is men or women whose experience of birth and parenting is out of step with their partner's. For example, it is her first baby but his third, or her second baby and his first. The combinations are complex and so, too, are the sensitivities of the people involved. Often, the shadow of former relationships hangs over this birth, 'Will she do the same as X?', 'Will I measure up to Y's performance?'.

If you have other contacts with the family, you may know the history of a particular couple. However, this information is often treated as secret, a reflection of how problematic many people find this pattern of parenthood. It can take several weeks for a couple to let the group know how this baby fits into their family and in the meantime you must, of course, respect their confidentiality. As always, don't make assumptions. Even in a group where everyone looks like the families on cornflake packets, there may be someone who faces these issues.

Couples in this situation may need extra encouragement to remember that each birth and each baby is completely unique. They may also need time to consider the effects of the new baby on existing children, who already face the additional complexities of belonging to a multiple family.

Classes for very young parents

Very young mothers (for us, that means under 18 years old) do not form a homogeneous group any more than do older women. Some may have such special needs that they need their own group. Others could benefit most by being treated in exactly the same way as any other expectant parent. Your approach may vary according to the numbers of teenage parents in your area, their willingness to attend existing classes, their particular needs and the issues they face.

The first step to take when considering your approach to teenage parents is to review your own attitudes and feelings. What do you really think about pregnant teenagers? Jot down your thoughts and impressions or talk them over with a friend or colleague (Chapters 21 and 23 suggests ways to do this effectively).

Does it make a difference to your feelings if they are married or in a stable relationship? Do you think that very young parents are:

- irresponsible?
- just getting pregnant in order to be housed?
- more likely to be promiscuous or to abuse drugs?
- incapable of being good parents?
- wrong not to have terminated the pregnancy?
- well advised to give the baby up for adoption?
- aware of the implications of their decision to have their baby and as keen as any parent to give their child the best and most loving care?

Most of these comments are opinions rather than facts and are, therefore, an unreliable basis on which to work. Some could be relevant to *some* teenagers in *some* circumstances. The important thing is to avoid assumptions and generalizations.

Teenage parents experience plenty of prejudice and difficulties and are likely to have fewer resources than their older counterparts. Whatever their background or circumstances, care needs to be geared to their individual needs *as they see them*, and offered with respect if they are to accept and benefit from it.

Integrated classes

The things women share when pregnant can more than balance out their differences. If they are treated equally and with complete respect, teenagers can benefit and gain confidence from being in a class with older women. One of us holds dear the memory of opening a session with the suggestion that the dozen or so pregnant women form pairs and tell each other the most surprising thing that had happened that week. This led to the memorable exchange between a 17 year old clad in leather telling her 'partner', a senior doctor, about reactions to her newly-shaved head only to have the doctor top that with her own two-day-old discovery that she was having twins. What keeps this memory alive is the fact that each one listened to the other!

Separate classes

However, these moments are rare and many teenagers do not come to 'ordinary' antenatal classes. If this is true in your area, it may make sense to run a course specifically for them. There are a few fundamentals to sort out before you start.

What kind of support do you have from your manager?

Unless your classes are closely linked to a clinic for teenagers or other medical check, it takes about two years for the grapevine to spread the word about your classes to potential customers. Until teenagers start coming because they have heard the classes are useful and non-threatening, you must set aside precious time for perhaps only a few takers. This is only possible with the rock-solid support of those in the hierarchy who allocate resources. Can you count on that kind of support?

Who will run the course?

The person who runs the class is the single most important determinant in whether a course for teenage mothers succeeds or flounders. Before you take on the job, ask yourself if you *like* working with this age group – not just can you do it, but do you positively enjoy contact with young women under 18? Can you consistently suspend judgement on those who may run their lives in ways very different from your own? If not, your job could be to find someone who would enjoy this challenge and to help them plan and run these classes.

What are your aims for the course?

If you work with teenagers, you are unlikely to cover the same ground as you might with older women. If you want to attract any group to classes and hold their interest, the content needs to be geared to their needs. So with teenagers you will probably find that you cover only one or two pieces of information per session that *you* feel are important. The rest of the time may be taken up with concerns that matter enormously to them, such as how to modify their clothes to accommodate a growing baby, housing worries, boyfriend troubles, parent troubles, or just plain chat and human contact. Some teachers find this frustrating and wonder how it squares with their professional expertise and training. Yet unless you let them take the lead, they will not come at all.

Where else can new parents go after your classes?

Many classes for teenagers welcome postnatal participation. New mothers gain confidence and self-esteem from sharing their experiences, and expectant parents learn from being with new babies. Also, the new mothers remain accessible for further help with parenting. This arrangement usually works best if it is limited to only a few months. After that time, the needs of young mothers with babies or toddlers are probably better met elsewhere. This can be a smooth 'graduation' if the next group exists and if the next group leader, too, has a friendly, informal supportive approach. Otherwise, you may find that mothers are reluctant to move on.

Have you thought about grandmothers?

The mother's mother often has as many concerns as her daughter. If you welcome both to your classes, the daughter may get little space for herself if her own mother either speaks for them both or uses the opportunity to address her own concerns. But excluding grandmothers, either by not inviting them or by running the group in such a way that they are not heard, could shut out the only support many young women have. In some places, teachers run open classes where all are welcome – grandmothers, partners, friends, older sisters. Sometimes, everyone meets together for common issues, while at others, they split into generation groups to consider pertinent issues and feelings with others 'in the same boat'. If you adopt such an approach, you will need to plan carefully either how you will brief each group to work without a leader or whether holding the classes with two or more teachers might make the arrangements easier (see Chapter 15).

What about very young fathers?

While it may be true that many pregnant teenagers are unsupported by the baby's father, there are some young men who are involved and concerned. How can you incorporate them and give them opportunities to find out about birth and parenting and talk about their concerns and feelings? Some of the suggestions in Chapter 17 are equally applicable here.

Designing a course for teenagers

It is important to make your sessions as far from school-type learning as possible, as many young women in an antenatal class will have only bad memories of formal learning. It often helps if a group meets in each other's homes or in a local youth centre, so that the antenatal teacher is their guest rather than the other way around. When asked for their comments about antenatal classes after their babies are born, teenagers usually cite the practical things: a tour where you see things and meet people, real babies to hold, bathe and soothe, or some of the activities suggested in Chapter 10. Antenatal teachers, too, have their

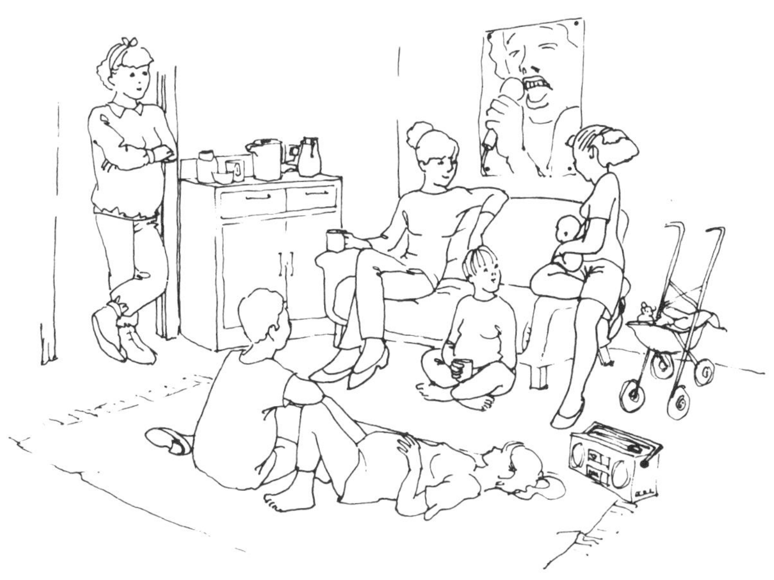

Figure 18.1

favourite ways of getting young women talking. Pop songs are good triggers to help them begin to sort out fantasy and reality when it comes to love and babies. Videos are less successful, although one sure winner is an episode from TV's *Eastenders* in which 'Michelle' gives birth in circumstances similar to their own.

When planning what to include in your course, be aware that you will probably be able to cover only a small amount of information and to try out only a few practical skills connected with giving birth. So choose the topics that really are the essentials.

That goes for changing lifestyle habits, too. It may be tempting to use the class as an opportunity for conveying health education messages, especially to those who smoke, drink or abuse drugs. However, this approach is likely to alienate people. Many people (and especially those in this age group) are very sensitive to anything that seems like bossing or telling off. Even your most important messages, therefore, must be carefully and tactfully conveyed. It is often far more effective to give wholehearted and genuine praise for any effort, no matter how small, that parents make to improve the health of themselves or their baby than to make them feel bad by pointing out harmful habits that they already know they have.

Working with teenagers is hard and sometimes heartbreaking. One experienced midwife said: 'It's what I like best because they *really* need me. The rest can get it somehow – books or friends or whatever – but for these girls, it's me or nothing.' You will need some equally powerful spur to keep going when you work with this group and you will also benefit from having time and assistance to review, let off steam and celebrate your successes. Part IV suggests ways to do this.

Meeting the needs of disabled parents

You probably will not think about how parents with a particular disability will manage pregnancy and parenting until you encounter someone who combines the two. Your first thought might be to gather information, starting perhaps with an appropriate pressure or self-help group. Some voluntary organizations hold registers of parents with various disabilities who are willing to talk with anyone who is similarly disabled. This link can sometimes be very helpful (see Appendix I). You could also read *The Baby Challenge* which gathers together general information about pregnancy and birth for disabled parents and offers a few pages of information on specific needs of people with some common disabilities (see Further Reading at the end of Part III). Finally, MIDIRS – the midwifery resource centre – holds a database of articles on disability and pregnancy (see Appendix I).

However, if you only consult these sources, you miss the most helpful and expert source of all – the person who stimulated your interest in the first place. He or she will often have done some research already and will surely know what is and is not helpful – so ask. This may be hard if you feel that, as the professional, you are expected to have all the answers already. However, people would much rather tell you themselves what they need and want. This puts them in control, maintains their independence and respects their knowledge and dignity. It also helps you to avoid mistakes and to be more likely to meet their needs.

Make sure that the questions you ask are genuinely open . . . 'How can Ted best adapt this position to hold you, Mandy?', rather than leading . . . 'Wouldn't you be more comfortable just sitting down for this bit?'. In a class, it may be difficult to balance a disabled person's need to be like everyone else (except in the few areas where he or she obviously needs extra help) with your desire to tailor what you teach to fit their particular situation. Check regularly that you are getting it about right, either as part of a more general feedback session or in a quiet aside during a coffee break or after the class.

As you work with a person who is disabled, keep reviewing your own attitudes and prejudices because these will seep into everything you do. Almost without exception, babies born to parents with disabilities are both planned and wanted. Can you welcome their decision? Those with physical disabilities are well used to devising ingenious ways of managing the demands of everyday living, so they will do the same in parenthood. Do you believe in their ability to care for their children?

Every parent will have more abilities than disabilities and even *dis*abilities are in some ways an asset. A mother in a wheelchair may not be very good at hide-and-seek, but she does have a lap always available. A deaf mother who uses sign language will have to work doubly hard to help her hearing child learn to speak, but her child will have two totally different ways of communicating and will be effectively bilingual. Can you see the benefits for the children as well as the difficulties?

The issue of attitudes to disability goes beyond exploring your own.

You may need to help parents with disabilities anticipate and find ways of coping with judgemental or unhelpful treatment during their pregnancy and hospital stay. By asking open questions of the group as a whole, you help everyone – not just disabled people – to plan for the aspects of hospital life they will find most difficult. Be careful about what you yourself suggest, because while one blind woman may welcome a sign over her bed saying, 'Please introduce yourself before you speak to me', another will hate the idea. Keep asking the parents what they would find helpful. They are the real experts in such matters.

Meeting the needs of parents from ethnic minority groups

Britain is a multicultural, multiracial society and many antenatal classes will reflect this reality. As an antenatal teacher, you need to be aware of cultural preferences and religious beliefs that parents in your group *might* hold without assuming any are, in fact, held in the group. When you work with any group, you need to demonstrate to parents

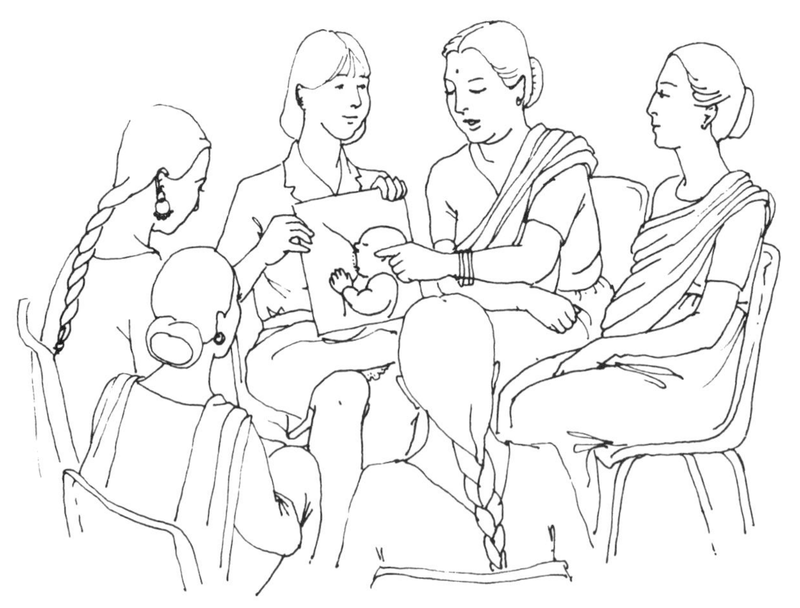

Figure 18.2

that you welcome diversity in all its guises – different ideas, different dreams, different ways of seeing the world as well as the different shapes, sizes and colours of the people present.

Sometimes, teachers find it hard to meet the needs of people from different racial or cultural groups within the class because they pretend they do not notice them. Acknowledging differences is contrary to the way many British children were raised. ('Don't point at that man in a wheelchair, it will embarrass him.'). You will be more effective as an antenatal teacher if you acknowledge differences. This helps people to talk about their ideas and beliefs if they wish and it allows the group to talk about racism and discrimination. There is overwhelming evidence that some ethnic minority groups regularly experience both. They might expect similar treatment from health professionals or from you in your class.

If you are white and were raised in Britain, you may need to read about and talk with people from other racial groups to discover that much of what you see as normal and acceptable is seen by black people as racist. You need to look at the language you use because words like 'black', 'Asian', or even 'British' will have strong connotations for some members of the group. Ask them what they would feel most comfortable with, then help others in the group to use the same terms. If you are white and British, make an effort to understand how it feels never to be allowed to belong. Are there experiences in your own life where you felt this? How would it be if that was an everyday experience?

Another awareness that will help you work with people whose culture differs from your own is to recognize how much of what we all do in everyday life is culturally determined rather than an expression of universal beliefs or values. If you are a white and British person who was raised in Britain, you may be as unaware of the rules, taboos and assumptions you follow as you are of gravity that holds you to your chair. Each of us, as a matter of course, makes assumptions about family life, about the role of men and women and about pregnancy, childbirth and parenting. In this country, it is generally considered 'normal' to have regular antenatal checks, to have a baby in hospital and to be cared for by strangers. The father is expected to be involved and to be present at the birth. Antenatal classes for many people are part and parcel of having a baby.

Many people do not share these beliefs. You can keep this idea in mind as you work with a multicultural, multiracial group. What might confuse or shock a woman who speaks little or no English or who cannot read? A woman who has had no experience of hospital and was raised in a place where she knew everyone by name and babies were born at home? One who views birth as women's work, entirely separate from the world of men? For people whose experience and expectations are very different from those of the majority, giving birth in this country can be alienating and terrifying. Even those with only slightly differing cultural backgrounds can become confused. One American woman, a trained nurse and veteran of nine months of antenatal care in England, expressed surprise that her baby was apparently delivered by a nun. The custom of calling senior nurses 'Sister' is unknown in the USA. How many more misconceptions can arise when people come from, for example, a non-western background?

By gathering the insights you need to answer questions like those in the last paragraph, then translating this awareness to the classes you teach, you benefit the whole group, not just individuals from ethnic minority groups. When you show you welcome diversity, you free up the whole group to share their thoughts and feelings. This approach helps parents of all backgrounds feel welcomed, respected and involved in what is happening in the class.

Learning about various ethnic groups

There are many ways to find out how people from cultures other than your own handle birth and parenthood. If there is a sizeable population of a particular group in your neighbourhood, locate and approach specialist advice centres and cultural associations. Ask your neighbours and workmates. You might learn from willing individuals who attend your classes, or consult the books listed under Further Reading at the end of Part III. You could also contact the King's Fund which maintains a database on individuals and groups working for improvements in services for ethnic minority groups. There is much to discover before you even know the right questions to ask, let alone what the answers might be.

As you gather information, bear in mind that not everything you learn about a particular ethnic or religious group will apply to any individual member of that group. People outside a culture often ask general questions like, 'What do Sikhs do about birth?', 'How do Filipinos feel about modesty?' or 'Do Orthodox Jewish men want to attend the birth?'. Tempting though such 'facts' may be, consider how would you react to the same kind of query about *your* group? How do the English feel about modesty? How do nurses feel about personal hygiene? What do mothers in Croydon want for their sons? You may be able to spot patterns or likely preferences, but you can never predict the answer for any individual.

Teaching to accommodate diversity

You will need to work out ways of explicitly recognizing any differences in the group without harping on them or making assumptions about cultural beliefs on the basis of race or skin colour. You can do this from the first moment of meeting as a group, perhaps starting by suggesting they find a partner and discover two things they have in common and two they do not share. Later, when discussing, for example, what they find hard or easy about going to antenatal clinics, you might bring up the issue of assumptions they meet that are surprising or disturbing. This may be an issue for people of different racial groups who have been brought up in the UK because, although they are perfectly familiar with British culture and British ways of giving birth, this is not always acknowledged by those caring for them. Still later, you could ask an open question about how they wish to greet their baby. This may vary depending on the parents' ethnic group. Some greet the baby with a special prayer; many practising Hindus welcome their baby to the world by putting honey on its tongue. What do the parents in *this* group want for their baby? Later on, you could help the group list the many ways that extended families might be involved in the first few days.

Another way of tailoring your class to the sensibilities of those present is to reconsider the content of your course. Women born and raised in India or Pakistan speak with horror of watching birth films with other women's husbands present. This ordeal has, some say, become a sort of initiation trial to be endured – they know it's coming and they steel themselves for it. This is hardly education. How could you achieve the aims you hold without embarrassing and humiliating some people in the room? In the same way, you could decide to include a topic – say circumcision, if that is likely to be an issue with the group. Orthodox Jews will probably have views about circumcision, as will some Gentiles and most antenatal teachers! How do you feel about it? How would you discuss it if an Orthodox Jewish couple was in the group?

Teaching physical skills, too, *might* require tact and discretion. For example, how would you teach touch relaxation or massage if you have an Orthodox Jewish couple in the class? Many Orthodox Jews do not wish to touch each other in public; often, husbands do not touch their wives during labour once the waters have broken. Remember that you will only know what the couple in your class want by checking with them.

If you have several people from the same group in your course, it may be helpful to offer them time together while the rest of the class focus on another topic. Alternatively, you might offer them a session on their own to discuss the specific issues that are important to them. This has the additional advantage of offering *you* a deeper insight into their needs and perspectives. In all these initiatives, make sure that you balance your concern to give each person scope for exploring their differences with your commitment to help every individual in the group feel a part of everything that is happening.

Separate classes

If parents from minority groups do not come to existing classes or if you have several who do not speak much English, a separate and specifically designed course may be the answer. However, before you begin planning for separate classes, take some time to try to discover why particular groups do not come to the ones you are already running. Could it be they do not know about them? Word-of-mouth publicity will only reach those similar to people you already teach. Handouts and brochures only work for those who can take in information in this way and who can read English. Local radio spots or announcements in public meetings could work, but are they targeted specifically at under-represented groups? You may even need to make yourself known to the perceived leaders of the community who will, in turn, pass your invitation on to others.

Perhaps people do not come because they cannot see the benefits of classes. The whole idea of groups getting together to learn may seem strange. Learning about *birth* in groups may be inconceivable to people who are used to finding out such things from relatives or neighbours. Many see medical people as healers, not teachers. How can you help them get a clear idea of what is on offer? The best people to help are those with one foot in each culture – yours and theirs. If you find such a bridge, look after the person well – he or she is not only your best asset, but also likely to be under great pressures and demands from both sides.

Another reason for not attending classes aimed at all pregnant women is the feeling that the classes are not for them. Perhaps under-represented groups feel your classes ignore certain issues or over-emphasize others. If this is so, you might decide to redesign your course to make it more accessible and relevant to the various groups in your community. Your revised plan will probably be an amalgamation of what you consider important, based on your own expertise and what you have discovered is likely to be relevant to the parents you hope will attend.

It is not always easy to accept the plan that is best for *them*. It may be hard to give up certain topics or approaches that seem to work well with other groups or that you consider to be the 'right' way to prepare for birth or raise children. But your job is not to make this group of people more like you, it is to help them feel confident and prepared for the experience of giving birth and raising healthy children. As with all groups, you will need to listen to parents, identify their needs, find out about their preferences and norms, then adapt what you do and say accordingly. Once you have run one course, their feedback will be invaluable in changing and adapting the next one.

This 'suck it and see' approach means you will need extra time and resources. This is an important point to raise with your manager. You will probably find working this way tiring and, at times, stressful. It will take more time to prepare and to recover afterwards. This isn't because these are 'problem people', but because you lack the certainties of shared assumptions. Working with other ethnic groups is a bit like your first driving lessons – nothing comes automatically. Remember how tiring that was? But in time, you drove without undue effort. The same will be true of the sensitive, creative work you do with people from cultures other than your own.

Working with interpreters

If you and your group do not share a common language, you will have to rely on an interpreter or link-worker in one of several ways. You could work as a team, each offering what you do best. In some places, the antenatal teacher acts more as a consultant, helping the link-worker gain the knowledge and group skills needed to run the class, then standing by as a resource for technical questions and ongoing support. Or you might feel a clear separation of roles is best, with you leading the group and the interpreter acting simply as the bridge between you and them. The danger with this last approach is that you will not have a full understanding of people's needs and responses and may not meet either fully. Most people do a bit of each of these ways of working in the space of a whole course.

Working well with an interpreter or link-worker requires skill, patience and a good deal of practice. Many books offer guidelines for good practice and one is suggested under Further Reading at the end of Part III. All of them agree that the key element in an effective working relationship is a clear understanding of what each of you wants from the other. Guidelines elsewhere in this book on team-teaching (see Chapter 15) may be helpful here, too.

You may have read the last paragraph about interpreters with a wry smile, thinking, 'If only we had one . . .' or remembering an instance when someone came to a group with very little knowledge of English. It is hard to see how you can offer real help when you do not share a common language. However, people frequently understand far more than they can express so you can convey a few messages if you are careful in the way you use English. Again, Further Reading lists a book we have found helpful in developing the skill of using English well with those who understand it with difficulty.

When you are trying to communicate with a non-English speaker, keep watch on your feelings. If you start to feel frustrated or desperate, chances are the other person is feeling this way, too. Instead of ploughing on or resorting to mimes that nearly always miss the mark, you might consider what else you can offer. A non-English speaker may benefit from simply being there with others. If the class takes place in a hospital, she has an opportunity to become familiar with the place in which she will give birth. A look and a smile that says, 'I'd like to communicate . . .' actually does. Or the person could take away written material for someone to translate for her at home.

Working with people from different cultural or religious groups than your own is challenging. It can also be very rewarding, since those who fit least easily into standard classes are the ones who could probably benefit most from contact with a teacher who really listens, is open, adaptable and regards it as a privilege to learn about their needs.

Other groups with a shared need

In any group there might be two or three people with a common experience such as having their first baby by caesarian section, an IVF conception, or single parenthood. It is almost always helpful to find occasions when they can work together either in discussions or on practical matters. This will cause no disruption if your group is used to breaking into smaller groups in a variety of ways for a variety of reasons.

Sometimes, there will be enough people with one experience to form a group tailored specifically to their needs. Some have already been mentioned in this chapter. Other examples we know about include groups for parents having twins, those adopting a baby, and those expecting a baby after a stillbirth or neonatal death. In these groups, you may have to work very hard to balance needs which resemble those of any other antenatal group with the addition of the special concerns that bring them to this particular class. Open questions and good feedback will help the group, and a chance to talk these matters over with a non-judgemental colleague will help you work well. Part IV of the book suggests ways to do this.

The concept of consulting parents may seem inadequate and some teachers find it very frustrating. They want the answers, not the questions! Of course you will need more information to work well with special groups or individuals with special needs. It will help to review the literature held in a resource bank like MIDIRS (see Appendix I) or consult the appropriate self-help group. Technical know-how will allow you to answer questions and anticipate likely issues. But you do not need to become an expert. What parents in special interest groups need is the chance to talk, listen, laugh and sometimes cry together, secure in the knowledge that the others really do understand. In time, that will include you, too.

19

Handling difficult topics

Ask any group of antenatal teachers what they find hardest to talk about in classes and you will get a varied list combining personal bugbears with topics that nearly everyone finds hard to handle. In the latter group, teachers mention sex, stillbirth and handicap and usually add cot death and postnatal depression. In addition, someone nearly always brings up the problem of giving accurate, balanced information on potentially controversial topics such as the use of intervention and technology. Which topics would appear on your list of difficult things to discuss with an antenatal group? What makes you or the parents in your group anxious?

This chapter suggests ways of dealing with topics that make you uneasy. If the ones we discuss don't match your own particular worries, concentrate on the approach – we hope it will be effective whatever the issues are for you. Of course, there are no promises that reading the chapter will make things easy. But with a bit of effort, some planning and practice, you can talk about them just as you do about other topics that are part of your course.

Reviewing your own attitudes

How do you handle difficult topics at the moment? Many teachers develop their own coping strategies. A few avoid some or all of the issues mentioned at the start of this chapter altogether, either because the topic is hard to handle or because there seems little point in worrying expectant parents about things that will probably never happen. Others say they are willing to cover anything, provided that it is brought up by someone in the class. Some ensure that certain subjects are always included unless a situation arises in a particular class which leads them to adapt their usual practice. What do you do?

In your antenatal course, do you include some or all of the boxed topics?

	Always	*Never*	*Sometimes*
Birth options (i.e. home birth, mobility throughout labour)			
Disadvantages and side effects of technology and interventions			
Disadvantages and side effects of drugs			
Sex during pregnancy			
Sex after birth			
Stillbirth or neonatal death			
Neonatal intensive care			
Cot death			
Postnatal depression			

How did you arrive at your decisions to include or exclude these topics? To think carefully about your reasons, try asking yourself the questions in the next box.

- What is (or what could be) my purpose in including or leaving out this topic?
- What information do parents have a right to know?
- What information might parents find helpful?
- Would my including this topic, even briefly, be honest?
- Would it enable parents to deal more effectively with events?
- Do the advantages of discussing this topic, even briefly, outweigh the disadvantages?

It is worth remembering that, even if you decide to exclude certain topics from your course plan, sooner or later they will be raised by a participant. Giving some thought to how you will respond when this happens will be time well spent.

Talking about sex

Many of us shy away from talking openly about sex. We may be unsure of our ground or afraid that others will be embarrassed or offended. This reticence is not surprising since, despite the apparent liberation of the 1990s, sex is still surrounded by secrecy and taboos. It may simply feel too risky to raise such an emotive topic. But if you shy away, is it for your benefit or for theirs?

What do parents want to know?

Most people have questions about sex they would like to ask, but don't. Many are glad to know that, barring obstetric problems, sexual intercourse is safe throughout pregnancy, neither damaging the baby nor triggering a labour that is not already imminent. Some people want to be more sexually active during pregnancy and others lose interest, sometimes completely. This can be true of both men and women and can cause major stress if partners are out of step with each other. The group may find it helpful to know that these reactions are common and that talking things through and understanding each others' feelings can help.

Information about sex after a baby's birth is fairly thin on the ground, but many women report they are uninterested in any sexual activity. Vaginal intercourse in particular can be problematic, perhaps because of exhaustion, soreness after stitching or slow return of natural vaginal secretions. Some new mothers feel too absorbed with their relationship with the baby to make space for their partner's needs.

New fathers describe changes, too. Some are put off by what happened at the birth or by changes in their partner's body. Many are afraid of causing pain. Most couples say it takes time, gentleness and understanding to resume any kind of active sex life. It is often a long time before anything like pre-baby sex returns.

If your class doesn't provide this information, where else will they learn it? Being informed can help parents avoid or minimize problems and anxiety. We find this a persuasive argument for including talk about sex in antenatal classes. You may not include the same information as that described above, but what will you offer to help parents cope with the effect of pregnancy on sexual relationships?

How and when to discuss sex

One way of offering information is to display books and leaflets which deal with sex during pregnancy and after the birth. Some useful ones are suggested in Further Reading at the end of Part III. If these can be borrowed or bought, participants can acquire the information they need or augment the information you have given. However, written material does not appeal to everyone. Those who are not used to learning through reading or who are reluctant to be seen borrowing such a book will have to rely on you.

Once you have decided on the information you think important to include in your course, think through the vocabulary you will use with the group (see Chapter 8 for general suggestions about appropriate language). Practice what you want to say by talking out loud or using a tape recorder. You may not want to go as far as the antenatal teacher who sat in front of a mirror saying 'penis' over and over again until it felt all right, but what *can* you do to release embarrassment and reduce awkwardness? The more confident and relaxed you are in your approach, the more receptive and open your class members will be.

Next, think through where it is logical to include talking about sex in your course. Covering sex in pregnancy is little use towards the end of the course when the women are about to give birth. Nor will the idea of sex after birth seem relevant if you include it in early classes. There are, however, lots of appropriate openings. For example, when teaching pelvic floor exercises right at the beginning of the course, you could mention practising during sexual intercourse – 'if you are still making love . . .'. If the class members make a list of changes in pregnancy, you could say, 'What about sex? Any differences?' as the group works through the lists. Towards the end of the course, you may spend time on the changes parenthood brings or lead a discussion on contraception. Whenever you bring it up, drop in references to sex rather than launching into a long information-giving session. Keep it light and be guided by their level of comfort and curiosity. Once you break the ice by mentioning sex, they might, too.

Talking about stillbirth and neonatal death

Death has been described as the twentieth century taboo and talking about stillbirth is particularly hard. Since it happens to only about one woman in a hundred, there may seem little purpose in raising the issue, especially as many antenatal teachers worry that they are creating anxiety where it doesn't already exist. In reality, almost all expectant parents have either thought or dreamt about this possibility, although few voice their fears. While it is true that they become subdued when stillbirth is mentioned, people later say it was helpful that the unmentionable was given a voice. It is the only topic we have ever been thanked for including in the course!

What information might be helpful

Apart from acknowledging the reality of stillbirth, there are certain pieces of information parents say are helpful. Notice that the statements below – unlike most of what you say to the group – are deliberately *not* directed at the listening parents.

> Most stillborn babies look healthy and as though they are asleep. Seeing and holding the baby, whatever its looks, can be very helpful. The reality of the baby's appearance is almost always better than the fantasy, and having time to meet and then say goodbye to their baby helps parents to come to terms with their loss. It gives them precious memories.
>
> It's routine in many places for the staff to photograph the baby so that parents can have a copy, either straight away or at any time later.
>
> Naming the baby and perhaps arranging a funeral can also help parents acknowledge and grieve their loss.
>
> Support networks are available for both parents. Fathers grieve, too, and need as much support as mothers.

Expectant parents can only hold a few thoughts about stillbirth because they are so distracted by their emotions. Pare down what you say to the absolute essentials.

How and when to discuss stillbirth

There are several ways in which stillbirth can be raised either by developing your own openings or staying alert for any the group offers. For example:

- Through newspapers, radio and television stories – stillbirth is often in the news.
- In a 'safe pot' exercise (see page 89) – you could join in the exercise and decide to introduce the subject.

- In a general discussion on reactions in the first few minutes after birth.
- Any time women mention dreams. Many pregnant women (and some men) have very vivid ones like dreaming the baby was dead or born able to walk and talk. You can comment that it is common for people to dream that something is wrong with the baby and that most of us have that fear buried somewhere. It's also worth mentioning that thinking or dreaming about stillbirth or abnormality does not signify that anything is wrong nor does it cause it to happen!

If you want to introduce the topic of stillbirth, you will find a way, but however well you time the introduction and however sensitively you handle what happens next, discussing stillbirth is depressing and the atmosphere in the class always becomes quiet and heavy. It's important to acknowledge this and then to ensure that there is plenty of time to lighten the mood and regain a sense of proportion before the class ends. Here are some points to keep in mind:

- If you bring it up, do so in the first half of a class and in the first two-thirds of the course.
- If someone else brings it up and you cannot handle it well, perhaps because you lack the time, then acknowledge the speaker and promise to find a place for it next week. Then be sure to fulfil your promise.
- Follow the discussion with a change of mood, either by doing something lively and practical (not relaxation which some find hard after this sort of discussion) or by discussion on some everyday topic such as baby equipment, choosing names or what to take into hospital.
- You may want to ask the next week if there are any repercussions from what was said the week before.

When a baby dies

Although stillbirth and neonatal deaths are uncommon, they do happen and are always shocking and hard to accept. If someone in your class has a baby who dies, you yourself will need support. You will also need to decide what support you will offer the bereaved parents. Finally, there is the decision as to whether and how the rest of the group will be told.

Parents whose babies are stillborn or die soon after birth often feel they have failed. They may associate you only with positive outcomes and healthy babies and feel that they are no longer entitled to your attention. However, your acknowledgement of their status as parents who have suffered a real loss can be very helpful, whereas your withdrawal is likely to accentuate their feelings of failure. You will need to work out what you can offer and ensure that you get time to deal with your feelings both before, and after, you offer your support, perhaps using a format like that suggested in Chapter 23.

You will then need to think through how to approach the rest of the class. If you teach open classes it may not be obvious that someone is missing, but if you teach a closed class or hold a reunion, the absence of class members is bound to be noticed. Will you wait until somebody asks or will you break the news to them yourself? Some teachers think it is better not to tell the rest of the class unless someone asks, especially if they have not yet had their babies. They argue that it will only raise anxiety and distress. Others feel the opposite, finding it is easier for everyone if the teacher decides when and how to break the news, as someone is bound to ask or find out sooner or later.

One compelling reason for telling the class is the benefit bereaved parents can feel when their group offers sympathy and support. Again and again, parents whose baby has died say that people avoid them, do not acknowledge their loss and treat them as though they have never been parents. By raising the matter publicly, you actively model a more sensitive way of helping those whose baby has died, and thereby add to the whole community's ability to handle tragedy more sensitively.

Whatever course of action you decide on, it is important to discuss it with the bereaved parents. They will have views and their privacy and feelings must be respected.

If you do tell the class, it is better to do it first thing and break the news as simply as possible. The amount of detail you give will depend on the bereaved parents' wishes. Allow time for people to assimilate the news and perhaps talk in twos or threes about how they feel. One way for the group to express sympathy is to send a joint card, signed by everyone in the class.

Some groups will need a long time to mull things over, others will want to move on more quickly. You will need to judge how long to give them. Then follow on by putting this sad event into proportion. Help them see that stillbirth is uncommon and the chances of it happening are small – possibly linking it to everyday risks like riding in a car which is far more risky for small babies and children. Afterwards, choose an activity that will lighten the atmosphere, although it is probably unrealistic to expect to send everyone home feeling happy.

This will have been a hard class to lead, so afterwards get some support for yourself before you go on to your next task. If you can arrange this in advance, so much the better.

Another time when you could help the class work through their feelings about stillbirth and neonatal death is when someone in the group describes a previous birth that ended in tragedy. You may know about this, discover it at the same time as the rest of the group, or even find out after the course has finished. If the parents share their experience spontaneously, you can help the group and the parents in all the ways already described – by listening while they tell their story, by encouraging others to share their feelings upon hearing the news, and by lifting the atmosphere when you judge it to be appropriate.

Sometimes, parents tell the teacher about a former pregnancy that ended in death or handicap but ask that it be kept from the rest of the group. Of course, they have the absolute right to remain silent, but occasionally this decision does affect the group in that the others sense that something secret is going on. This can make them both anxious and unwilling to share their own thoughts and feelings freely. In some cases you may want to explore with the bereaved parents why they wish their experience to be kept secret. We believe an antenatal class may be one of the best places to help parents see this shocking event as part of the wider reality of giving birth.

Talking about birth options, technology and intervention

Antenatal teachers vary considerably in their approach to discussing birth options, medical interventions and obstetric technology. It's not just antenatal teachers who have polarized views, parents have them, too. The people who come to your class will hold a whole cross-section of attitudes about how babies should be born, about the role of technology in pregnancy and labour, and how involved they themselves want to be in the decision-making process. Many expect the medical professionals to make decisions and are surprised that others want to be involved when there are 'experts' to do it for them.

A few are determined to maintain control of what happens to them at all costs and are suspicious of (or downright hostile towards) any advice they are offered. A common middle way is to be interested in a handful of choices, concentrating on getting them 'right' and taking a more passive approach to the rest.

The job of the antenatal teacher is to help all these people, from the ones who question nothing to the ones who question everything, to become more flexible and open minded. That's the best hope they have for making really good decisions. Seeing only one side of any issue is liable to leave people disappointed or disillusioned. Just occasionally, polarized views lead to serious battles between carers and parents or teachers and hospitals. If two-way communication breaks down, unnecessary risks may be run or there may be avoidable confrontations between parents and health professionals.

Antenatal classes can make a real difference if the teacher doesn't join in the polemics but stands back, offering as full, balanced and accurate information as she can. This isn't easy. If you work in a hospital setting where choice is limited by standardized care and the use of technology is routine, you may feel it unwise to include discussion of the drawbacks of non-medical induction, routine monitoring, artificially ruptured membranes or even mundane matters like the mythical benefits of salt baths. The argument goes: 'If that's what is in store for parents, why make it harder for them?'

On the other hand, you may believe so strongly in natural birth and be so aware of the disadvantages of technology and obstetric management that you find it hard to give appropriate time to discussing them at all, let alone their benefits. This argument goes something like: 'If everyone else is extolling their virtues, why should I add to the hard-sell?'

Or you might be so accustomed to high-tech birth that you simply can't see why anyone would want a physiological alternative. 'Would you have your appendix out without anaesthesia?'

Of course, these views are more like caricatures than reality. Most of us fall somewhere between these extremes. Where do you fit? Can you be as open minded as you would like parents to be? Unless you can, you will not offer parents the help they deserve to help them face what may be difficult choices.

Taking the middle road is not the same as sitting on the fence. It means knowing your hobby-horses and deciding not to ride them. It means paying close attention to what you say and how you say it. It means offering parents ways of making the best decisions they can given *their own circumstances, beliefs and experience*; then accepting that their views may not in any way resemble yours. It can't be done without regular fresh looks at current evidence and regular assessments of your own beliefs.

Assessing your personal views

If you find it hard to talk calmly and objectively about any topic, find a sympathetic listener and think out loud about your own experience and feelings. We know people who have done this about home birth, their relationships with medical people, the decision about breast- or bottle-feeding and even seemingly trivial matters like dummies. Although one person's straightforward choice is another's 'red rag to a bull', the pattern of introspection remains largely the same. Ask yourself:

- What do parents have a right to know about the use, advantages and disadvantages to the mother or to the baby in this matter?
- What am I *not* saying? Why? What am I *stressing*? Why?
- What's the basis for the information I give? My own belief? Traditional practice? A review of the research literature? The word of a powerful figure in the field? Or what?

You might find it helpful to list the pros and cons of the topic or issue, check on any relevant research data or find out about the approaches other teachers use. Then review your approach. You may find it useful to discuss your views and feelings with a supportive listener, decide what changes you want to make and how you will do this. Part IV of the book is all about these issues.

Taking time to identify the subjects you find hard, then to work through your own attitudes are two steps towards making your teaching more effective. However, you and the parents you teach are not islands. Whatever you do as an antenatal teacher is bound to be influenced by the situation in which you work and by the routines where the women you teach give birth. This is the focus of the next chapter.

20

Being an agent for change

In the last chapter we discussed topics that teachers commonly find hard to handle because of their personal feelings or because the subject is viewed by society as embarrassing or charged with anxiety. This chapter is about difficulties that arise because of the system in which a teacher works or in which the people she teaches are cared for. Sometimes, institutions create problems for the teacher, especially those who aim to teach for choice, as described in Part I.

Over the past few years, staff in many units have been at great pains to assess all their procedures, with a view to reducing the amount of routine intervention and offering parents real choices. Even in units where this is not so, communication between staff and parents has become more consumer-friendly, so that individual mothers may feel they are given good reasons for the treatment they receive. Despite the smoother communications between parents and carers, anyone with an overall view – and that includes antenatal teachers – can see in some places that local practices are out of step with what parents are promised during antenatal care or with national standards of good practice as outlined in reviews like *A Guide to Effective Care in Pregnancy and Childbirth* (see Further Reading at the end of the Chapter.

There are at least two ways of tackling the problem of the gap between what parents want (or are promised) and the care they actually receive. Some antenatal teachers see the best solution as helping and encouraging parents to make choices outside 'the standard package' if that is what they want. Others favour changing the system that puts pressure on parents and teachers to accept the routines and procedures regardless of personal attitudes and beliefs. Of course, many teachers who want to see changes do a bit of both.

Helping parents make their own choices

It is almost inevitable that you will discuss various options for managing pregnancy and birth if you teach people who are attending different hospitals. As parents discuss what they themselves experience, it soon becomes evident that there is no absolute or correct way of managing pregnancy and birth. By encouraging discussion that acknowledges this variety, you will probably find that talk flows almost inevitably to weighing up pros and cons. To be helpful, this awareness of differences will need supplementing with more practical skills. Parents need help to move from having their own views to communicating them to their carers. The books on assertiveness listed at the end of the chapter could point you to useful techniques.

You can encourage the same weighing up of choices even if everyone in your group will be managed in the same way. You do this by treating *all* decisions – not just the ones involving obstetric management – as a choice between two or more valid options because that's what most of them are. What are the pros and cons of staying home in early labour? Of having an alpha fetoprotein (AFP) test? Of having your partner present for a scan? Of an epidural anaesthetic for a caesarian? Of having a home birth? Of dummies? Parents soon get used to this approach and may themselves apply the same criteria to decisions about more clinical matters like drugs, induction, monitoring and immunization. You can respond to queries with current research, but make sure it is drawn from the widest possible spectrum of evidence. As you do, you reinforce the notion that there is very rarely a right or wrong, just choices between various consequences, some positive, some negative.

Another way to put decisions about technology in context is to point out how many decisions parents make hour by hour and day by day that directly affect their baby. This is an integral part of parenthood and it is something they will be expected to do for years after the baby is born. Some expectant parents need help to see that they are already doing so. This helps them put choices about intervention and technology into proportion. Their confidence to make choices often grows when reminded how successfully they have managed so far.

Taking personal responsibility for initiating change

Some antenatal teachers are dissatisfied with the kind of approach described in the last few paragraphs. They say it puts too great a burden on parents themselves to be good decision makers, skilled negotiators and assertive communicators. Why not make the system one that can cope with parents' choices? . . . one that really offers informed consent? . . . one that allows for differences of opinions and differing needs?

Taking an active role in causing change may feel more alarming than changing things indirectly through parents, but with planning and patience it may be possible to raise issues so that those in authority are prepared to listen. There are several strategies you might use to be an effective agent of change and only you can decide which are appropriate for you and the situation in which you work. You may have, yourself, discovered a way that works. Here is one we have tried and tested.

Identify the key issues

If several aspects of the care parents receive make you uneasy, it is tempting to want to tackle all of them at once. However, choosing one issue helps you focus your attention and allows you to discover which strategies work and which do not. Make your first efforts on whatever issue will be least threatening to those that might resist. If you already have colleagues who share your view, you can discuss with them what to tackle first.

Identify potential allies

You are less likely to get discouraged and more likely to succeed in raising awareness of issues (if not in precipitating actual change) if you work with at least one other person. He or she needn't be someone in a position of authority nor someone you work with closely. By asking others open questions and listening attentively to the ensuing discussion, you raise awareness, learn about different perspectives and perhaps discover who shares your views. Slowly, you might build up a group of people who are also prepared to question an attitude, practice or procedure.

Gather evidence

Try any or all of these things:

- Formalizing the evidence you get from parents in your classes (see Chapter 21).

- Doing a literature review. Although many practices haven't been evaluated, there is a growing body of research on many routine obstetric procedures.
- Talking to staff from other hospitals and to independent midwives.
- Approaching local branches or the national offices of the relevant voluntary organizations such as the National Childbirth Trust (NCT), Maternity Alliance, Professional Association of Childbirth Educators (PACE), or the Association for Improvements in Maternity Services (AIMS). Each will have feedback from its members. (Addresses are listed in Appendix I.)

  In all these efforts, the way in which you and anyone who works with you approaches people makes a difference. You might find it helpful to check on assertiveness techniques (see Further Reading at the end of this chapter). Then practise what you will say and, just as important, how you will say it.

Next steps

When you have identified the issue, gathered some support and marshalled the evidence, take time to review. It may be that by merely raising the issue and encouraging people to think afresh, things start to change and nothing more needs to be done. Or you may conclude that the time is not ripe for taking things further. Every now and again there are 'windows of opportunity' when change and review are easier to initiate because it is already happening – for example, when a unit moves to a new location or two units merge, when protocols are reviewed, when training programmes are revised or when a team approach to care is being planned. However, these are not always good times for you to add new issues. If the change is causing large amounts of stress or extra work for staff or managers, then one more change may be the last straw.

If you judge the time is right, you have several options. Among them are to:

- approach the relevant manager or person in authority to discuss the issue and present your evidence;
- propose a local review, a trial or a consumer satisfaction survey;
- ask the local Maternity Services Liaison Committee to review the issue;
- raise the matter with the local branch of the Royal College of Midwives or Health Visitors group.

What other approaches could you try in your unit?

Precipitating change is not easy, especially if you do it from within a hierarchy. It can take an inordinately long time to see results and the going is bound to be tough somewhere along the way. The support of at least one other person will make a real difference. Regularly take time to review then reassess the situation and adapt your plans in the light of what you are finding out. You may not succeed the first time, but you will certainly learn something about how to initiate change.

Further reading

The International Standard Book Number (ISBN) is given where possible and should be quoted when ordering the book from your bookseller.

Preparing for parenthood

Auckett, Amelia (1988) *Baby Massage: The Magic of the Loving Touch,* 2nd edn, Thorsons, Wellingborough (ISBN 0-7225-1793-9)

Chamberlain, David (1987) The cognitive newborn: a scientific update. *British Journal of Psychotherapy,* **4**, 30–71

Jessel, Camilla (1988) *Joy of Birth*, Methuen Children's Books, London (ISBN 0-416-01572-7) [Full of black and white photos of new babies.)

Jessel, Camilla (1990) *Birth to Three,* Bloomsbury, London (ISBN 074-750-5195) [Lots of realistic photos to get discussions going.]

Nilsson, Lennart (1990) *A Child is Born,* Doubleday, London (ISBN 0-385-40085-3) [Fascinating photos accompanied by explanatory text]

Rankin, Gwen (1988) *The First Year of Life: How to Adjust to Your New Baby,* Piatkus, London (ISBN 0-861-88739-5)

Verney, Thomas and Kelly, John *The Secret Life of the Unborn Child,* Sphere, London (ISBN 0-7221-8821-8)

Wambach, Helen (1982) *Life Before Life,* Bantam, Toronto (ISBN 0-7221-8821-75)

Working with fathers

Balaskas, Janet (1984) *Active Birth Partners' Handbook,* Sidgwick and Jackson, London (ISBN 0-283-99038-4)

Beail, Nigel and McGuire, Jacqueline (1982) *Fathers' Psychological Perspectives,* Junction Books, London (ISBN 0-86245-083-7)

National Childbirth Trust (1982) 'Becoming a Father', a NCT leaflet – see Appendix I

Roeber, Johanna (1987) *Shared Parenthood: A Handbook for Fathers,* Century, London (ISBN 0-7126-0724-2)

Seel, Richard (1987) *The Uncertain Father,* Gateway, Bath (ISBN 0-946551-26-X)

Groups with shared needs

Campion, Mukti (1990) *The Baby Challenge: A Handbook on Pregnancy for Women with a Physical Disability,* Routledge, London (ISBN 0-415-04859-1)

Friedrich, Elizabeth and Rowland, Cherry (1983) *The Twins Handbook,* Robson, London (ISBN 0-86051-214-2) [A book for parents.]

Hewitt, Patrica and Rose-Neil, Wendy (1990) *Your Second Baby,* Unwin, London (ISBN 0-04-440608)

Linney, Judy (1983) *Multiple Birth: Preparation – Birth – Management,* Wiley (ISBN 0-471-25849-0)
Mares, Penny, Henley, Alix and Baxter, Carol (1985) *Healthcare in Multiracial Britain,* National Extension College – see Appendix I (ISBN 0-860-826139)
National Childbirth Trust (1982) 'Some Feelings of Disabled Mothers', a booklet published by the NCT – see Appendix I
Redshaw, Margaret, Rivers, Rodney and Rosenblatt, Deborah (1985) *Born Too Early,* Oxford Medical Publications, Oxford (ISBN 0-19-261542-4) [A book on premature babies.]
Shakeman, Jane (1984) *The Right to be Understood: A Handbook on Working with, Employing and Training Community Interpreters,* National Extension College – see Appendix I (ISBN 0860-82-4691)
Sharpe, Sue (1987) *Falling for Love: Teenage Mothers Talk,* Virago, London (ISBN 0-86068-841-0)

Handling difficult topics

Bing, Elizabeth and Colman, Libby (1977) *Making Love During Pregnancy,* Bantam Books, London (ISBN 0-553-01079-4)
Buckman, Rob (1988) *I Don't Know What to Say,* Papermac, London (ISBN 0-333-46983-6)
Enkin, Murray, Keirse, Marc and Chalmers, Iain (1989) *A Guide to Effective Care in Pregnancy and Childbirth,* Oxford Medical Publications, Oxford (ISBN 0-19-261916-0)
Henley, Alix and Kohner, Nancy (1991) *Guidelines for Professionals: Miscarriage, Stillbirth and Neonatal Death,* Stillbirth and Neonatal Death Society – see Appendix I (ISBN 86990-315-3)
Inch, Sally (1985) *Birthrights: A Parent's Guide to Modern Childbirth,* Hutchinson, London, available from the National Childbirth Trust – see Appendix I (ISBN 0-09-146031-X)
Inch, Sally (1985) *Approaching Birth – Meeting the Challenge of Labour,* Green Print, London (ISBN 1-85425-024-8)
Kitzinger, Sheila (1985) *Women's Experience of Sex,* Penguin Harmondsworth (0-14-007348-5)
Kohner, Nancy and Henley, Alix (1991) *When a Baby Dies,* Pandora, London (ISBN 004-440-5669)
National Childbirth Trust (1988) 'Sex in Pregnancy and After Childbirth', a leaflet published by the NCT – see Appendix I
Panuthos, Claudia and Romeo, Catherine (1984) *Ended Beginnings: Healing Childbearing Losses,* Warner Books, New York (ISBN 0-446-32956)

Being an agent for change

Bond, Meg (1988) *Stress and Self-Awareness: A Guide for Nurses,* Heinemann, London (ISBN 0-433-03490)

Dickson, Anne (1982) *A Woman in Your Own Right,* Quartet Books, London (ISBN 0-7043-3420-8) [An accessible introduction to assertiveness.]
Lindenfield, Gael (1986) *Assert Yourself,* Thorsens, Wellingborough (ISBN 0-7225-1558-8)
Peters, Thomas and Waterman, Robert (1982) *In Search of Excellence,* Harper and Rowe, London (ISBN 0-433-03490)
Phelps, Stanlee and Austin, Nancy (1985) *The Assertive Woman,* Arlington Books, London (ISBN 0-85140-731-5)
Plant, Roger (1987) *Managing Change and Making it Stick,* Fontana Collins, London (ISBN 0-00-636873-5)

Part IV

Thinking about you and your teaching

21

You and your teaching: self-assessment and skills assessment

In good antenatal classes, parents change, learn, enjoy themselves and benefit in a host of other ways. It is, of course, rewarding to whoever runs the class to watch these things happen. But they don't come for free – you give your time, your attention and your energy in order to meet parents' needs. If you are to remain effective you, too, need time and attention. It's like looking after your bank account – if you don't make deposits, there will be trouble.

Start with yourself

Finding time may seem difficult, but caring for yourself is just as important as caring for the people who come to your classes. You, too, need time for relaxation and the chance to let off steam. Even if your feelings tell you otherwise, you need and deserve opportunities to recharge your batteries by doing something you enjoy whether it is music, gardening, painting, swimming, reading or hill-walking. There are many ways of keeping your 'bank balance' healthy. What matters is that you have time for *yourself*. If this seems hard, think about talking it through with someone who can listen while you decide what you want to do then encourage and support you in doing it.

Think about your teaching

As well as looking after yourself, you need to nurture your teaching skills, update your information, review your attitudes and feelings, and assess and improve your skills. After teaching for a while, most of us feel the temptation to run on autopilot. Resist this by regular reviews of what you do and how you feel about it.

Think over what you teach, especially any topic or activity that you find boring or difficult to handle objectively. The questions in the box (or others you devise yourself) might help.

- What do you find hard?
- What gets in the way of your doing it effectively?
- What have you been told, seen or experienced in the past about this particular topic/activity?
- How is past experience influencing you in the present?
- Is this influence relevant to your present-day situation?

Pay attention to small doubts and niggles as well as the larger ones that leap to your mind. Through exploring them, you will gain self-awareness and you may even trigger some new enthusiasm or fresh insights about parts of your course that have lost their sparkle.

ASSESSING YOUR SKILLS AND EFFECTIVENESS

In order to go on being effective and continue to develop your skills, you need some information about how you have been doing so far. This may sound a pretty daunting prospect! Many of our memories of assessment, performance appraisal or feedback provoke winces rather than smiles. Have you been corrected in front of others, been told in great detail what you were doing wrong, or felt humiliated by criticism? Most of us have.

There is another way and, thankfully, school reports and training records now reflect the need to accentuate the positive. Constructive feedback and skilful assessment build on your successes rather than offer a dreary round of 'could do betters'. Not only does this feel less painful, it is also more effective. You are more likely to respond constructively to suggestions for improvement if you know clearly what you are already doing well.

Of course, not everything you do will be praiseworthy – none of us is perfect. But effective feedback follows a rough rule of thumb, whereby 80% of the time is spent looking at what you do well and 20% looking at what you could improve and how you could go about making these changes. However you review your skills – whether by self-assessment, by peer assessment, by asking parents, or by some other way you devise for yourself – you will benefit most if you stick to the 80:20 ratio.

Self-assessment

Many of us are quietly assessing ourselves most of the time. To extract useful information, rather than getting bogged down in what went wrong or having the same thoughts again and again, it helps to set aside a few minutes, perhaps at the end of a class, to use an informal procedure for self-assessment. Ask yourself:

- *What did I do well?* Nothing is too trivial! Acknowledging and welcoming a late arrival, remembering people's names, noticing that some people need further explanations of some aspect of labour, leading the relaxation at a slow gentle pace, ending the class on a warm note – these are all signs of your skill as a teacher. Acknowledge them.
- *How do I know?* Think about the effects of your actions – what signs were there that what you did was helpful? For example you might say: 'I know that taking a minute to welcome Sue helped, because she settled in and became part of the group straight away.' Or: 'I know that my explaining *x* in more detail helped because Mary said she found it clear and there was a look of understanding on other people's faces.'
- *What could I improve and how?* Resist the temptation to do this until you have extracted all the positive thoughts from the event. When you have identified one or two areas you want to improve, consider questions like: Where or from whom could I get input or help? What steps do I need to take to set this up? When will I take the first step?

An informal personal review need not take much time. You can either do it by yourself or, better still, talk it through with a friend or colleague. This is especially helpful when you are new to teaching or putting new ideas into practice.

Long-term review

After some time – say six months or a year – you might find it useful to take an over-all look at your teaching. This will be more effective if you have someone to assist you and to take some notes for you to keep.

Teaching review

- What are you doing well in your classes? Be very specific and detailed and give examples of the effects of each skill you identify. Nothing is too trivial.
- What skills have you improved – what new ideas have you incorporated since your last review?
- Outline any changes and improvements you have made to your course. If you set goals at your last review, take time to appreciate what you achieved.
- If you did not reach a previous goal, identify why.
- What have you found hard?
- What would you like to improve?
- What input or ongoing training have you had since your last review?

Forward planning

In the next 6 months/year:

- How do you see your classes changing or developing? For example, are there any organisational changes in the pipeline?
- What changes do you personally want to make to your classes?
- How exactly will you set about achieving these?
- What is your order of priority for these?
- What input or support do you need?
- Where and when could you get it?
- What is your first step?

Set a date for your next review

Your assistant's role is to listen, to keep you going and to remind you to be detailed and specific. She can ensure that you stick to the ratio of 80% successes to 20% improvements, and encourage you to celebrate your skills and abilities and to believe that you can develop still further. One way your assistant can help is to ask a series of questions, like those in the box opposite, then listen carefully to the answers, jotting down any useful information that arises.

Peer assessment

Another way of finding out how you are doing is to invite a colleague or interested friend to sit in on your class, possibly just once or through a whole course. Think carefully about who you choose, searching out someone who will be open and honest, someone who you trust and respect. Most of us have feelings of competitiveness or not being good enough. These feelings can be recognized, discussed and set aside, but if either of you holds them strongly in relation to the other, pairing up will probably not be fruitful. Your observer might start by reading through this chapter. Then you will need to do some careful preparation together.

Preparing for observation

You need to agree what she will be observing. She might observe the class as a whole, noting specifically what went well. Those with less experience as observers may find it easier to concentrate on one or two specific aspects of each class. Here are some examples of areas to focus on.

- *Your skills as a group leader* – is everyone included and involved? Is discussion usually channelled through you or is it bounced between participants?
- *The atmosphere* – is it relaxing and welcoming? Do participants relate well to each other?
- *Your appearance,* tone of voice and body language.
- *The pace of the class* – are participants interested and actively involved throughout the class?
- *Your ability to convey technical information* clearly and simply.
- *Your skill in teaching relaxation*, positions, massage and breathing etc.

- *Your ability to respond flexibly* to questions and issues that arise spontaneously.
- *Your skills in welcoming and involving fathers* and other supporters.
- *Your inclusion of the baby* as a real and sensitive individual.

Other issues also need sorting out before the class. Where will the observer sit? If she is straight opposite you, you will be constantly reminded of her presence and be tempted to focus on her. If she is out of your sight, you may worry about her reactions.

What will her role in the group be? Will she sit silently? Will she contribute when she wants or wait for you to invite her comments? What about taking notes, bearing in mind that others find it uncomfortable or distracting to have someone writing things down?

Preparing the participants

Anybody joining a group will change the dynamics. You have only to think what it's like when you begin to relax at a party, thinking all the guests are present, only to have the doorbell ring and you are required to make another adjustment. It is a bit like that when an observer appears. Participants need forewarning that someone else will be joining the class. Tell them why she is coming lest they wonder who is being observed or what is really going on! When the observer actually appears, introduce her, remind the group of her role, and perhaps do a round of names as you would do for any new arrival.

Reviewing the class

Whenever possible, arrange to talk about the class straight afterwards. The class will then be fresh in your minds and you are spared the trauma of waiting.

Receiving feedback

When you are offered feedback from your observer, the most important thing is to listen and accept what you hear. This is easier said than done. Curiously, it is usually particularly hard to listen to what went well and you may have to make a real effort to pay attention to positive feedback. If you find it hard to believe, or are unclear about precisely what you did well, ask for more detail. This is not selfish, big headed or boastful. Once you know, you can repeat good practice and grow in confidence.

Keep on listening when improvements are suggested. If you think these are valid, review with your observer the various ways in which you could achieve them. If you don't think a suggestion is valid, ask for more detail about what has been said. If you still find it hard to accept, check it out with someone else whom you trust to be honest with you. Should you then see the relevance, look for ways of improving. If you decide the observation is not valid, set it aside with the proviso that you might review it in the future, especially if someone else makes the same observation.

Giving feedback

Feedback is only useful if it helps the person you are giving it to. Constructive feedback focuses mainly on the positive and is most effective when it is detailed and specific. Giving facts is nearly always useful, whereas your personal views and opinions are unlikely to help the other person. If you can substantiate your comments with examples of the effects of the person's skills or actions, she is more likely to absorb what you are telling her.

It helps to focus on what the teacher did rather than on her personality or attitudes. It is easier to hear and act on, 'You show people you are listening by leaning forward and keeping eye contact', rather than, 'You are a caring person'.

When you are giving feedback about what might be improved, keep it to a minimum. Nit-picking is not helpful, so stick to the most important factors. Only comment on things she can actually change. For example, you may think smaller classes would benefit the participants, but the leader's manager may be adamant that it is better to have large classes than to exclude people.

If you suggest improvements, assist the person to think about how she might set about achieving them. If you suggest more than one, help her establish priorities so that the task feels manageable.

In all that you say, assume that whoever is receiving your feedback has been doing the best she can at present and that, with support, she is able to develop and improve her skills. People who have had the chance of working in this way remember the experience with satisfaction.

Feedback from parents

In recent years there has been a substantial number of studies to evaluate antenatal classes. Women respond in all kinds of ways during pregnancy, labour and the early days of parenthood and for all kinds of reasons. That is why it is hard to establish conclusive, objective data about the effectiveness of classes. Randomized controlled studies have shown that women who attend classes use significantly less analgesia during labour, although this reduction could be due to a variety of factors which are unrelated to classes. No other important effects of antenatal classes have been demonstrated – see *A Guide to Effective Care in Pregnancy and Childbirth* in the Further Reading list at the end of Part III. If you would like to know more about the studies that have been done, MIDIRS (see Appendix I) holds a comprehensive database.

Despite the lack of hard evidence, it is clear from the growing popularity of classes that parents want them and find them helpful. Although objective measures would be very useful, the subjective responses of parents are also important. If parents seek out classes and find them informative and supportive, and as a result become more confident and able to take responsibility for themselves and their baby, then the classes have served a valuable purpose.

So how can you find out about your classes? You can gain a certain amount of information by collecting and analysing numbers. How many women come to your class compared with the total number giving birth in the catchment area? If your classes still have available places, then seeing the proportion of childbearing women in attendance going up would be one sign of success. How many people come because of word-of-mouth recommendation? When that number rises, you know the 'grapevine' is saying, 'Her classes are good.' Look at how many people complete the whole course. Of course, there are many obstetrical surprises which could intervene but if many people attend erratically or drop out after a few classes it may be time for a rethink.

You could also count how many people want to come and can't get a place. Is the number rising? If demand far outstrips your ability to meet it, that may bring its own stresses, but it also satisfying to know that what you offer is what people want. If your analysis of numbers points to difficulties, find a supportive colleague with whom you can discuss the whole matter and decide how best to deal with what you've discovered.

Objective feedback like numbers and percentages may feel neat and solid, but subjective feedback offers many clues about what you are doing well and what needs improving. You are probably gathering these clues informally all the time. By observing the effects of what you do as you teach, you get an idea of what works and what needs review.

Participants may tell you they enjoyed the classes or found some particular aspect useful. Or you can gather an impression of how you are doing by inviting people at the end of the class to tell you one idea, or piece of information or skill they found particularly interesting or useful (see Chapter 6 for how to do a round). People often notice and appreciate things you are not even aware of or did not think particularly significant. You could also do a similar exercise at the end of the whole course.

Alternatively, you might do a more formal study of your classes by asking parents to fill in an evaluation form. This could focus on the classes themselves, or on what happened during labour or the first few days of parenting. If you choose to ask questions about labour or early parenthood, you need to be aware that other factors besides your classes will have influenced events.

What kind of form will you use? A very structured one which invites only yes/no answers is easy for the majority to fill in and straightforward to collate, but offers only limited information. You get richer responses and a new slant on what happened if you use headings or unfinished sentences to focus people's thinking on various aspects of the class, with plenty of space for their responses. However, people who are unused to expressing themselves on paper are unlikely to write much or enjoy the experience. A compromise is to combine the two approaches in a form containing predominantly closed questions with a few open ones at the end like:

- What did you enjoy most about the classes?
  'The thing I enjoyed most about the classes was . . .'
- What did you find most useful?
- What did you wish we had included or spent more time on?
- What improvements can you suggest?

The feedback you get is unlikely to be conclusive and will vary depending on when you ask for it. Will it be at the end of the last class of the course? After the course is finished? Immediately after the babies are born? Or even a few months postpartum? Waiting makes things more complicated because it involves mailing questionnaires, keeping track of the answers and chasing up people who do not respond. However, you might decide that it is worth taking the trouble now and again since asking for feedback after a certain lapse of time gives a clearer view of the real impact of your course.

Using the reunion

An excellent time for getting feedback is during what many people call a reunion. This is usually timed for a few weeks after the last baby in the group is due. Although participants will probably have their hands too full of babies to fill in forms, you can structure the session so that each person has an opportunity to tell the group about the birth and her or his experience of early parenthood. If you have a large class you may need to divide it up into small groups so that each person has time to tell their stories and be listened to. You can then ask each person questions like the open ones mentioned under the last heading (pages 171–172 have more suggestions about debriefing well).

Receiving feedback from parents

If you ask parents questions, you need to be prepared to accept *all* the answers you get. Sometimes, participants who appeared to enjoy the classes hugely and to gain support and confidence from them say afterwards that they didn't help much. Or someone will say about a topic you covered thoroughly, 'You never told us about *x*'. Sometimes the others say, 'Oh yes, she did' but if they don't, you need to accept the criticism/comment cheerfully or you might get no more feedback from this group! Many parents focus on the positive in order to avoid hurting the teacher's feelings, so you may need to encourage them to suggest improvements as well. Try asking, 'What would have made classes even better?' Telling them that their comments play an important part in helping you to ensure your classes continue to be useful to parents may elicit helpful feedback.

In conclusion

Inviting feedback takes courage, particularly if your previous experiences have been unhelpful. It is still worth while doing it, provided that you focus on your successes and plan for improvements rather than concentrating on mistakes and inadequacies. It is the best way we know of gaining confidence, and nurturing your ability to continue developing as an antenatal teacher.

22

Trying out new approaches

Discovering your own ideas

A few people seem to have an infinite ability to pull imaginative ideas out of their hats. A much larger number feel unable to innovate or incorporate new ideas. In reality, we all have a greater capacity than we realize to think creatively. Given the right circumstances, we can all innovate existing ideas and build on them. One vital element is the will and energy to have a go. That's where the comments in Chapter 21 about looking after your own needs come in. Unless you do, you won't keep alive the spark of creativity we all have within us.

To start thinking creatively, you must first catch your ideas. They tend to come unexpectedly, in the supermarket queue, first thing after waking or when you are doing something completely divorced from teaching. Because they come at inconvenient times and are probably incomplete, they get undervalued or ignored. Notice when and where ideas tend to occur to you and instead of letting them slip away, jot them down, however unworkable or inconvenient they seem.

Later, take time to play with them, exploring even the ones that appear ridiculous or impractical. Then develop your best ideas before you try them out. This process will work much better if you have an interested and attentive listener. You don't have to come up with complete ideas. This is an opportunity to think out loud, to explore and develop your ideas with the help of another person. You could do this informally or adopt a more formal procedure like the one suggested in Chapter 23.

Incorporating new ideas

In our work with health professionals and lay teachers we often offer them a new idea, show them something they've never seen before or suggest they read something inspiring. A few reactions are very common. 'I can't wait to try that!' 'I've got to go back to Square One and change everything!' 'However much I wanted to, I could never do that.' All these statements need some thought and moderation.

Whether you are unsure of yourself or eager to try out something new, you are likely to be more effective if you take one step at a time and do some thinking and planning first. So before you include anything new in your classes or reject a tempting innovation out of hand, think about the points listed in the box.

- Plan for one change at a time, and start with something that feels possible for you. In this way you can assess your effectiveness and build your confidence.
- Clarify your purpose in including this topic, exercise or approach. What do you aim to achieve?
- Examine your own feelings and attitudes to it.
- Explore ways others have handled it.
- Adapt these so that you use words and approaches that are your own.
- Try it out yourself. Use a tape recorder, a mirror or practise with a friend or colleague who can give you constructive feedback.
- Fit it into your course plan, linking it to other topics or using it as and when you judge it will be most useful for the group.
- Evaluate your effectiveness by observing the immediate effects and inviting feedback from parents.
- Assess usefulness by listening to parents' postnatal reflections.

Bit by bit, guided by the immediate and long term feedback you receive, you can develop or modify what you do. Given the choice between evolution and stagnation, most people have little difficulty deciding which they prefer.

23

Setting up a working partnership

It is perfectly possible to do many of the things we suggest here in Part IV on your own. However, you may find that you can think more clearly, solve problems more easily and review how you are doing more readily if you work with one or more other people who also want the chance to think and review. This kind of co-operative working doesn't just happen, it needs careful planning and structure.

You may already have a working partnership like this with one or more others. If you do, you will need no reminding of the benefits of talking things over and will know that it can be both satisfying and fun. If you have not experienced this way of working, you may want to try it out for yourself. Here we suggest one way to set up a working partnership that could help and support you as an antenatal teacher while you review your aims, assess your skills and effectiveness, develop your thinking and plan for the future.

Starting a partnership

To get started, think through the people you know, both colleagues and friends. They could be familiar with antenatal teaching or working in other fields. Who do you feel you can talk to? Who are the people you feel you could turn to when you need a hand? Then offer a clear invitation to one or more of them to set up a partnership where everyone – not just you – will benefit.

When setting up a partnership, the fewer things you assume and the more you spell out the better. Each partner needs to be clear and happy about the way you intend to work together. These issues are central:

- *Use of time.* Where will you meet and how often? What time of day is best and how long will you spend together? How long will the partnership go on for? Do you want to set up a trial period and see how things go? If you agree to be available to each other on the phone in between meetings, discuss when you would prefer not to be phoned (e.g. 'Not after nine' or 'Avoid weekends').

- *Confidentiality.* This is vital if you are to feel able to express yourself fully and freely. Each person needs to be certain that nothing she discusses with her partner(s) will be repeated to anyone else. This is taken for granted when clients are concerned, but is often forgotten when it comes to colleagues and friends.
- *Privacy.* You need a room where you will not be overheard, overlooked or disturbed by people, telephones or personal pagers. In most workplaces this is hard to find, but it is worth making an effort to ensure privacy.
- *Equal time.* Ensure that the time you spend together is divided so that each partner has an equal amount to use in whatever way she wishes. This division of time may seem artificial at first, but if you are not scrupulous about it, sooner or later one person will take more than the other(s). Of course, there will be times when one partner has a crisis or special difficulties and things get out of balance but everyone deserves a fair share of this valuable asset.
- *Respect.* Each of us deserves complete respect because each of us is doing the very best we can, given our current knowledge and circumstances. Appreciation and respect enhances our ability to clarify our ideas and think creatively. So even if you are listening to ideas that you think are ill conceived, it is important to maintain an attitude of non-judgemental respect *for the person* you are listening to.

  Respect also includes sticking to arrangements you make to meet or call each other, unless there are exceptional circumstances. If you phone unexpectedly, check that it is convenient and, if not, fix another time to talk. It is not helpful for either of you to try to talk and listen when distracted by other demands.
- *Competitiveness.* Feelings of competitiveness may creep in, especially if your partner is also teaching classes. If they are not dealt with, they can spoil the relationship and lead to problems. Usually, competitiveness arises when we do not feel good about ourselves, so it can be helpful to remind each other of the qualities and skills you each have. You may also need to come to an agreement about using or adapting each other's ideas. Who do ideas belong to? How can they be used for the benefits of the parents you teach, a goal you hold in common?

- *Trust*. Mutually trusting relationships are to be cherished. Clarify what trust means to each of you so that it can grow and strengthen as you work together.

Using your working partnership

Once agreements are clear – and that may take a while – you can turn to the task of helping and supporting each other. Again, fairly formal arrangements work best, although it may seem stilted or strange at first. When you meet, divide the time available equally, offering each partner a turn as speaker while the other(s) act as assistants and timekeepers. Where more than two people are meeting, it is a good idea to choose a primary listener, because it is easier to talk to one person. Those not actively involved in talking or listening should be focusing their attention on the speaker and listening in the same way as the primary listener. Everyone should have a turn at being the primary listener, so that each person can develop these skills as well as having time for themselves.

The speaker decides how she will use her time. She may want to work on some of the issues we have already discussed. Alternatively, she may simply need to let off steam or talk through a personal problem.

Being an effective working partner

Listening

A working partner's main function is to listen with complete respect. You show this by looking approving and friendly, relaxed and attentive. Good listening also means setting aside your own ideas and thoughts and instead, focusing entirely on what your partner is saying and doing. This is easier said than done, because stray thoughts creep in, along with the urge to give advice or tell her what you think. Whenever this happens, resist the temptation to intervene and firmly set your own thoughts aside. With practice, you will find it gets easier to keep your total attention on the speaker.

As a listener, you do not need to find solutions, give answers, advice or reassurance. With your attention and approval, the speaker will solve her own problems, develop her own thinking and reach her own conclusions. Assume that she is not only a clear capable thinker but the best person possible to deal with the issue she is tackling. Encourage her to take risks and to say the things she might be thinking but be too shy or embarrassed to talk about. If you don't, her best thinking or the most important issue might be missed.

Asking questions

One way of helping people develop their thinking and awareness is to ask an open question. Questions should be used sparingly and be carefully thought out. They should move people on in their thinking and only be asked for the benefit of the speaker, not because you, the listener, would like to know the answer. *When it is relevant* you could ask a question to help her

- *Develop and clarify her own thinking:* 'How else could you do this?' 'If you did it your way, what would that be?'
- *Talk about her feelings:* 'When that happens, how do you feel?'
- *Explore links with past experiences:* 'Does being in that situation remind you of anything?' 'What was it like for you then? How is it different now?'
- *Overcome feelings of inadequacy or bypass blocks in her thinking:* 'If you assumed that you knew exactly how tackle this – what would you be saying, what would you be doing?'
- *Prioritize:* 'What is the most important factor, or the first thing to tackle?'

Building on success

When we are aware of our strengths and abilities, we feel better and find it easier to try out new things. At the start of her time, encourage the speaker to talk about what has gone well since you last met. These do not have to be momentous happenings. Small successes or positive events at work or at home are fine.

If she feels unable to tackle something, let her know you believe she can deal with it and remind her of things she has done well in the past. A good way to end her turn is to tell her something you genuinely like about her or have learned from her.

Offering support

There may be occasions when the speaker needs to deal with her feelings before she can think clearly. If someone is angry, frustrated, sad or scared they will need to release these feelings first. You can help by having a relaxed, supportive and encouraging approach to a speaker who wants to express her anger, shake off her fears or simply needs to cry. If this is what she needs to do, that is the best possible use of her time.

Managing your working partnership

In order to ensure that your partnership continues to be useful to each partner, build in time to discuss what is going well and what could be improved. It is useful to do this at the end of a trial period and then every few months.

Plan time for having fun together. This may seem incompatible with your overall purpose, but laughter loosens tension and revitalizes the links between you. You'll get more out of your partnership if you mix play with work.

If there are more than two of you and anyone leaves, the working relationship changes. Rather than letting these changes just happen, why not end by celebrating the time you have had together? When the person has left, acknowledge the differences and develop the partnership in whatever way seems appropriate.

Similarly, the partnership changes when someone new joins. If the rest of you have worked closely together for some time, you will need to work out ways of including and integrating the newcomer. She may need to know about the history of the partnership and how you have worked in the past. She will certainly need to know about the commitment and any ground rules you have set, such as confidentiality and sharing the time equally. It is also important to take her views and needs into account rather than expecting her to slot into your established system.

At some point, however fruitful and enjoyable your partnership has been, it will end. It is better to make a positive decision to end than to let it grind to a halt. You can then celebrate the time you have had together. Tell each other what you have enjoyed about the partnership and about each other and end on a creative and positive note.

In conclusion

The ideal kind of partnership is an oasis where you can be yourself, where you don't have to get it right and where it feels safe to take risks. You can express your feelings, pick yourself up when life feels tough and be reminded of your strengths and qualities. It is also a place to celebrate successes, however small, and somewhere where you can laugh and have fun.

When you make time for your own needs, either with others or on your own, you nurture your effectiveness as a teacher and yourself as a person in all the areas of your life. Our own families, work and friendships have been strengthened when we practise for ourselves what we suggest here for you. We hope yours will be too.

24

Ongoing training

Alhough we can all develop new ideas and, if we keep our eyes and ears open, come across interesting and innovative developments, most of us need more systematic input from time to time. That means planning and organizing ongoing training. Here are some ways you can ensure regular chances to keep up to date and abreast of developments. We recommend that you use several, so that you encounter a broad range of opinion, information and techniques.

Teachers' meetings

The best meetings occur regularly and are large enough to bring together different ideas yet small enough to allow people to get to know each other. Most combine a chance to chat and share news, with a review of a specific topic chosen by the group. Many have regular 'case reviews', where individuals bring to the group particular issues or difficulties that arose in class. The good thing about teacher groups is that they are relatively informal and close to home, so you have the best chance of considering issues relevant to your own circumstances.

Teacher groups that go on being useful and lively are the ones that take time to look after themselves *as a group*. They spend time on ground-rules, commitment, their common goals and regular reviews of how things are going. The group process will be somewhat different from that described in this book because most teacher groups have no designated leader. If you are interested in the dynamics of groups without a designated leader, or want some insights should your teacher group run into trouble, the books on groups in the Further Reading at the end of Part II may help the whole group focus on the issues.

Some teacher groups make a real effort to build bridges between those who work in statutory services and those in the voluntary sector.

Sometimes, links grow slowly over many years, starting cautiously with shared lunches and informal chats designed to decrease suspicion and increase the sense of shared purpose. In some places, there are regular lively meetings where participants learn from and value the contributions of everyone else regardless of where they work.

Workshops and seminars

There is a wide and growing range of events lasting from one day to a week or more. You can find out about ones connected with antenatal education through professional journals, hospital bulletin boards, voluntary organizations or informal networks.

You will also gain a great deal from workshops less directly related to antenatal education. How about courses that look at the process of teaching and communicating such as assertiveness training, adult learning, groups and groupwork, counselling techniques or bereavement counselling? Then there are more content-based courses like those describing alternative and complementary medicine, offering the latest views on postnatal depression or state-of-the-art technology in special care. You will never keep abreast with all that is happening but keeping in touch in even a few areas will enhance your sense of competence and relevance. None of us enjoys feeling 'left behind' and it can seriously undermine your confidence.

Many of the topics mentioned in the last paragraph can be tackled through distance-learning packages. The Open University has literally hundreds of courses which you can do at home. The National Extension College (see Appendix I) has a more limited but nevertheless useful catalogue of topics. Polytechnics and colleges are rapidly developing ways for mature students to tap into continuing education, both in health studies and across the whole curriculum. If you have one nearby, ask for their prospectus and enquire about their efforts to improve access and distance learning.

There is, of course, a fairly constant struggle between the training people want and the resources that are needed to provide it. One way to get the most of the little that is available is to share what you learn with your teacher group or in a report-back seminar with other colleagues. PROSPECT workshops are very cost-effective, as they bring in trainers rather than sending people away in ones and twos. You save travel cost and you enhance the chances of applying new ideas on the job if a number of people train together.

Books, leaflets and magazines

Birth and babies, as one publisher told us, is one market that will never be saturated. The result is a steady flood of books and magazines on the shelves aimed at pregnant women/couples and a smaller output aimed at their carers. Much of it is repetitive or a passing fad, but you need to keep an eye on what is new. Ask parents what they are reading and how they feel about it. Check out reviews in professional journals and take time for an occasional browse at your local bookshop or newsagent.

Look out for books that keep on being mentioned or that seem to be taking on the mantle of an enduring reference book or key text. These are probably worth reading, either on your own or as part of a group. Some of the ones we have found of lasting value are mentioned in this book and you may also have your favourites. If you find a book you particularly like (or dislike!), why not pass it around and suggest a lunchtime discussion with a few friends or colleagues. Another possibility is to ask your teacher group to devote one meeting now and again to books, asking everyone to read a different one, then tell the group about it.

The consumer perspective

Reading the books that expectant parents read is only one way to keep in touch with consumers. Various voluntary groups publish in-house journals and several issue leaflets and pamphlets for free or very little cost (see Appendix I for names and addresses).

Just keeping track of existing organizations and what they set out to do is a big task which happily you can leave to others. MIDIRS (see Appendix I) keeps a database on voluntary groups and sells a directory of organizations relevant to childbirth that is updated annually.

Radio, television and newspaper coverage

The media provide a window on voluntary organizations and consumer perspectives, although you need to keep in mind that the ideas and views are filtered through the journalist who wrote the story. Some teacher groups run a kind of informal cuttings service where everyone watches for and saves what they see and hear. This is a good way to spot trends, identify new worries or fears among parents, and to discover charismatic people or innovators. You need this kind of input to keep your classes topical and relevant.

Often, the problem is not finding out what consumers are thinking but of keeping your own attitudes and feelings on the back burner long enough to take in what they are saying. Childbirth evokes strong emotion and deep conviction and you will find much that is contentious, 'far out' or different from your viewpoint. However, you cannot offer parents the balanced information they deserve to make the best choices for *them* unless you explore as wide a spectrum of thinking as possible with as open a mind as possible. One teacher of firm views found her own way: 'I think of it as detective work and my job is to gather the clues. . . .'

And finally . . .

At the end of each antenatal course, the parents you have been working with leave. You have given them information, passed on skills, offered them opportunities to review their attitudes and feelings and to discuss them with each other. Now they must handle their own individual experiences of labour, birth and parenting in their own unique ways.

You may have great hopes for them or perhaps some fears. You probably wonder did they enjoy the classes or were they just being polite? Will they remember anything you have taught them? Perhaps they won't find anything useful at all. Whatever your feelings, it is now up to the parents in whom you have invested so much. They will accept or reject what you offered. They may use information and skills in ways you have not thought of. The ways things work out for them may be very different from anything you envisaged. So the end of the course heralds a new beginning for parents and your role becomes peripheral. Ultimately it is now up to them.

We, the authors of this book, now find ourselves in a similar position. We have spent many months writing and focusing our attention on the needs of antenatal teachers. We have set out our ideas and approaches and tried to prompt reflection and reassessment. However, in reality, this book is merely a launching pad. Now it is up to you. Have fun and enjoy your teaching as much as we have.

Appendix I: Addresses of organizations

ACTIVE BIRTH CENTRE
55 Dartmouth Park Road, London NW5 1SL (tel. 071 2673006).
Runs antenatal workshops and yoga based exercise classes. Holds conferences and workshops.

ASSOCIATION OF CHARTERED PHYSIOTHERAPISTS IN OBSTETRICS AND GYNAECOLOGY (ACPOG)
c/o The Chartered Society of Physiotherapy, 14 Bedford Row, London WC1 4ED (tel. 071 2421941).

ASSOCIATION FOR IMPROVEMENTS IN THE MATERNITY SERVICES (AIMS)
21 Iver Lane, Iver, Buckinghamshire SLO 9LH (tel. 0753 652781).
Offers information, support and advice to parents and health professionals on all aspects of maternity care. Produces a quarterly journal.

ASSOCIATION OF RADICAL MIDWIVES. (ARM)
The Coppice, 62 Greetby Hill, Ormskirk, Lancashire L39 2DT (tel. 0695 572776)
Supports those having difficulties in either giving or receiving good maternity care.

BLACK HEALTH UNIT
57 Charlton Street, London NW1 1HU (tel. 071 3833841).
Aims to redress the problems faced by black and minority groups regarding health care.

BLISS-LINK
17–21 Emerald Street, London WC1N 3QL (tel. 071 8319393).
Supports parents with babies in special care and bereaved parents.

CAESAREAN SUPPORT NETWORK
2 Hurst Park Drive, Huyton, Liverpool L36 1TF (tel. 051 4801184).
Offers information on all aspects of caesarean delivery and one to one counselling.

CRY-SIS
BM Cry-sis, London WC1N 3XX. (tel. 071 4045011).
Offers self-help phone support for mothers with crying and sleepless babies.

EXPLORING PARENTHOOD
Latimer Education Centre, 194 Freston Road, London W10 6TT (tel. 081 9601678).
Runs workshops for parents to encourage them to find their own ways of coping with their problems.

HEALTH EDUCATION AUTHORITY
Third Floor, Hamilton House, Mabledon Place, London WC1H 9TX (tel. 071 3833833).
Disseminates information on health promotion issues and supplies leaflets, posters and resource lists.

HOME BIRTH CENTRE
Flat 3, 55 Elm Grove, Southsea, Hampshire P05 1JF (tel. 0705 864494).
Offers information and support to those considering a home birth.

INDEPENDENT MIDWIVES ASSOCIATION (IMA)
94 Auckland Road, London SE19 2DB
Provides continuity of care for women having a home birth.

JOINT BREASTFEEDING INITIATIVE
Alexandra House, Oldham Terrace, London W3 6NH (tel. 081 9928637).
A joint initiative between the Breastfeeding Promotion Group of the National Childbirth Trust, the Association of Breastfeeding Mothers and La Leche League, to improve support for breastfeeding mothers.

KING'S FUND CENTRE
126 Albert Street, London NW1 7NF (tel. 071 2676111).
Holds information on health services, planning and organization. Runs conferences and workshops.

MATERNITY ALLIANCE
15 Britannia Street, London WC1X 9JP (tel. 071 8371265).
Campaigns for improvements in rights and services for parents and babies. Publications list available.

MATERNITY LINK
Old Co-op, 42 Chelsea Road, Easton, Bristol BS5 6AF (tel. 0272 558495).
Provides support, advocacy and, if desired, English tuition to antenatal and postnatal non-English speaking women.

MIDWIVES INFORMATION AND RESOURCES SERVICE (MIDIRS)
Institute of Child Health, The Royal Hospital for Sick Children, St. Michael's Hill, Bristol BS2 8BJ (tel. 0272 251791).
Publishes a quarterly compilation of articles and research for midwives. Provides database searches on individual topics. Also publishes a comprehensive list of organizations in *The Directory of Maternity Organisations* (ISBN 0-9514241-2-2).

MULTIPLE BIRTHS FOUNDATION
Queen Charlotte's and Chelsea Hospital, Goldhawk Road, London W6 0XG (tel. 081 7484666 ext. 5201).
A professional organization which supports parents of twins, triplets etc. Provides specialized advice to professionals and the public.

NATIONAL ASSOCIATION FOR STAFF SUPPORT (NASS)
9 Caradon Close, Woking, Surrey GU21 3DU (tel. 0483 771599).
For Health Service employees.

NATIONAL CHILDBIRTH TRUST (NCT)
Alexandra House, Oldham Terrace, London W3 6NH (tel. 081 9928637).
Runs a national network of antenatal classes, breastfeeding classes and postnatal support. Runs training courses for the above and study events for health professionals. Publications list available. Produces a quarterly journal.

NATIONAL CHILDBIRTH TRUST (NCT) PARENTS WITH DISABILITIES GROUP
Purvisdale, 11 Spennithorne Road, Flixton, Manchester M31 2DF (tel. 061 7481970).
Offers a contact register of parents with disabilities for mutual support.

NATIONAL EXTENSION COLLEGE
18 Brooklands Avenue, Cambridge CB22 2HN (tel. 0223 316644).
Publishes books and learning packages for adults. Catalogue available.

NIPPERS
c/o The Sam Segal Perinatal Unit, St Mary's Hospital, Praed Street, London W2 1NY (tel. 071 7251487).
Provides information on prematurity and sick newborns. Encourages the setting up of parent-to-parent support groups.

OPEN UNIVERSITY
PO Box 188, Milton Keynes, Buckinghamshire MK7 6DH.
A huge range of short and degree-producing courses. Ask for the most recent prospectus.

PARENT NETWORK
44–46 Caversham Road, London NW5 2DS (tel. 071 4858535).
Offers parent support and education groups.

PROFESSIONAL ASSOCIATION OF CHILDBIRTH EDUCATORS (PACE)
107 Eynsham Road, Botley, Oxford OX2 9BY (tel. 0865 862124).
Accredits and supports childbirth educators and provides basic and further training.

PROGRESSIVE AND INNOVATIVE PARENTCRAFT TEACHERS SUPPORT AND INTEREST GROUP (PIPSI)
Pine House, Ransome Hospital, Rainworth, Mansfield NG21 0JB (tel. 0623 22515 ext. 4661).
Aims to make parentcraft teaching fun and informative for teachers and expectant parents. Publishes activity pack – cost £8.50 + £1.45 pp.

PROSPECT
4 Kiln Lane, Headington, Oxford OX3 8EX (tel. 0865 62537).
A partnership of experienced educators who design and run workshops for health professionals on a range of topics, including antenatal education, communication skills, stress management and team-building.

ROYAL COLLEGE OF MIDWIVES
15 Mansfield Street, London W1M 0BE (tel. 071 5806523).

SCOTTISH CRY-SIS SOCIETY
24 Greenhill Avenue, Griffnock, Glasgow GH6 6QX (tel. 041 6388602).
Like Cry-sis offers self-help phone support for mothers with crying and sleepless babies.

SCOTTISH PREMATURE BABIES SUPPORT GROUP
5 Sidlaw Drive, Wishaw, Scotland (tel. 0698 356074).
Offers one-to-one support.

STILLBIRTH AND NEONATAL DEATH SOCIETY (SANDS)
28 Portland Place, London W1N 4DE (tel. 071 4365881).
Offers support and befriending to bereaved parents. Members available as speakers. Publications list available.

SUPPORT AFTER TERMINATION FOR FETAL ABNORMALITY (SATFA)
29–30 Soho Square, London W1V 6JB (tel. 071 4396124).
Offers individual and group support to parents who have undergone termination of pregnancy for abnormality. Publishes booklets and pamphlets.

TWINS AND MULTIPLE BIRTHS ASSOCIATION (TAMBA)
59 Sunny Side, Worksop, Nottinghamshire S81 7LN (tel. 0909 479250).
Gives encouragement and support to parents with twins, triplets or more. Holds a register of Twins Clubs which offer informal support and friendship.

TWINS AND MULTIPLE BIRTHS ASSOCIATION SCOTLAND (TAMBA)
3 Park View, Kilbarchan, Renfrew PA10 2LW (tel. 05057 4622).
See TAMBA.

TWINS AND MULTIPLE BIRTHS ASSOCIATION BEREAVEMENT SUPPORT GROUP
32 Denton Court Road, Gravesend, Kent DA12 2HS (tel. 0474 567320).
Parent-to-parent support for bereaved parents who have lost one or both twins, or one or more triplets or quads.

Appendix II: Visual aids addresses

Catalogues

Visual aids catalogues are available from:

ASSOCIATION OF CHILDBIRTH EDUCATORS (ACE)
148 Hereford Street, Forest Lodge, New South Wales 2037, Australia

CHILDBIRTH GRAPHICS LTD
1210 Culver Road, Rochester, New York 1409–5454, USA (tel. 0101 212 716482 7940).

NATIONAL CHILDBIRTH TRUST MATERNITY SALES LTD
Burnfield Avenue, Glasgow G46 7TL (tel. 041 6335552).

Pictorial teaching aids

In addition to the above sources, you can get charts and drawings from:

GREEN PRINT
10 Malden Road, London NW5 3HR (tel. 071 2673399).
Thirteen charts (30 x 42 cm) of the illustrations in Sally Inch's book *Approaching Birth* (see Further Reading at the end of Part III).

PICTORIAL CHARTS EDUCATIONAL TRUST
27 Kirchen Road, London W13 0UD (tel. 081 5679206).
Sixteen charts on childbirth (35 x 50 cm) – cost £21.60.

Cheap paper for charting

Approach the office of your local free newspaper and ask for the end of rolls of newsprint.

Index

Acting, 138–139
Active learning techniques, 82–94
Agenda for classes, 45, 50–52, 164
Analogies and metaphors, 67–68
Assessment of teaching, 209–218
  in team-teaching, 149
  and working partnership, 221–226
Attention span, 54
'Attitudes and feelings' topics, 32, 34, 37

Baby, emphasis on, 158–159
Birth, life after, *see* Parenthood
Birth options, 20, 195–197, 198–199
'Block-and-push' technique, 120
Body language, 63–64, 73
  as visual aid, 133–139
Booking system, 31
Books and magazines, keeping up to date with, 229
Breastfeeding: as a topic, 32, 56
Breathing, 114–121
  linking relaxation to, 106–107
'Buttons', 93

Changing the system, 198–202
Charts: as visual aids, 144
Choice, teaching for, 21–22
Closed groups, 29–31
Closed questions, 73–74
Colour-coded cards, 35–38
Communication, 63–70
  through interpreter, 185–186
Compliance, teaching for, 20–21
Conclusion-drawing activities, 86–88
Confidentiality, 49
Contractions, modelling, 119–120, 138–139
Co-operative working
  team-teaching, 101–102, 147–151
  working partnership, 221–226
Courses, training, 228

Demonstration
  by teacher, 133–139
  with visual aids, 139–145
Description, accurate and realistic, 69–70
Diagrams: as visual aids, 144
Disabled parents, 178–180
Discussion, 71–81
  of 'difficult' topics, 188–197
  fathers and, 167–168
  problems with, 77–79
  starting of, 73–76, 88–89
Doll, teaching, 139–140
Drawing activities, 88–89
Dreams, 193

'EastEnders', 178
Embryo, models of, 140–141
Emergency delivery, 165
Emotions/emotional topics
  and group discussion, 79–80
  and open/closed groups, 29, 30
  and pregnancy, 7–8
  and relaxation exercises, 110
  and subgroups, 48
Encouragement and affirmation, 15
Ethnic minorities, 46, 90, 180–186
Euphemisms, 67, 68–69
Evaluation form, 217–218
Excretion, talking about, 67
Exercises, 131–132
Expectations of antenatal classes, 9, 10–11
Experienced parents, 170–173

Family members, 8
  substitutes for, 10
  of teenage parents, 176
Father(s), 8, 161–169
  language and, 65, 166
  physical skills and, 122, 123, 166–167
  sex and, 190
  teenage, 177

Feedback
  from observer, 214–215
  from parents, 216–218
Fetus, models of, 140–141
First meeting, 42–43
Fitness during pregnancy, 131
Friends and colleagues (of parents), 8

Groups(s), 27–31
  active learning in, 83
  closed, 29–31
  discussion, 71–81
    fathers and, 167–168
  getting started as, 43–47
  information from, 59–61
  open, 27–29, 31
  seating arrangements of, 41
  subgroups and, 47–49, 72
  teachers', 227–228
  team-teaching and, 147, 150

Handouts
  information from, 58–59
  publicity with, 39–40
Health information, 18–19, 178
'How to Catch a Baby in the Kitchen', 165

Information, 53–62
  activities to check and reinforce, 85–88
  communication of, 63–70
  from group, 59–61
  inaccurate, reshaping of, 60–61
  topics, 31–33, 37
  use of, 61–62
Intervention, medical, 195–197

Labour
  breathing for, 114–121
  positions for, 96, 125–130
'Labour Line', 87–88
Language, 64–69
  and experienced parents, 171
  and fathers, 65, 166
  and physical skills teaching, 104–105, 115
Latecomers, 42–43
Leading questions, 74
Leaflets
  information from, 58–59
  of other organizations, 229
  publicity with, 39–40
Learning, 12–16, 53
  active, 82–94
  past experiences of, 11
Lectures, 54–57
Lifestyle changes, 7–9
  see also Parenthood
'Lucky dip', 90–91

Massage, 121–124
Media, consumer information from, 229–230
Medical terminology, 66–67
Men *see* Fathers
Metaphors and analogies, 67–68
Mime, 134
Multiple familes, parents with, 173

Names, learning of, 45–47
Neonatal death, 193–195
New ideas, 219–220
  sources of, 227–230

Observer, assessment by, 213–215
Open groups, 27–29, 31
Open questions, 74–75
Ordering activities, 85

Panic, breathing against, 118–119
'Panic stopping', 109
Paperchase, 60
Parent-centred classes, 21–22
Parenthood, preparation for, 157–160, 172–173
  activities related to, 89–93
Partner *see* Father
Partnership, working, 221–226
  see also Team-teaching
Peer assessment, 213–215
Pelvic floor exercises, 131–132, 191
Pelvic rocking/tilting, 132
Perineum, model of, 141
Persuasion, teaching for, 18–20
Photographs, as visual aid, 143
Physical change, 7
Physical skills, 95–132
  ethnic minorities and, 184
  experienced parents and, 171
  fathers and, 122, 123, 166–167
  topics, 31–34, 37
Placenta, models of, 140, 141
Planning of course, 27–38, 164, 171

Posters
  information from, 58, 144
  publicity with, 39
Postnatal
  invitation to parents, 159, 168–169
  reunion, 218
  see also Parenthood
Posture, 125–130
  linking relaxation to, 107
Priority sheets, 92–93
Problem-solving activities, 86
Publicity, 39–40, 164, 184–185

Questions
  from participants, 15
  from teacher, 73–76
Quick relaxation techniques, 109–110

Recognition activities, 85–86
Relaxation, 100–112
'Relaxation ripple', 110
Respect and acceptance, 14, 50
Reunion of class, 218
Room for teaching, 14, 40–41
  and practising physical skills, 96–97
Rules, 49–50, 77

'Safe pot', 89
Second and subsequent babies,
  parents expecting, 170–173
Self-assessment, 209–210, 211–213
Seminars, 228
Sex
  talking about, 67, 190–191
  touch as alternative to, 124
Slide-shows, 144, 169
Smoking, advice on, 19
Special needs, people with, 170–187
Stillbirth, 191–195
Strong feelings, in group discussion,
    79–80
Subgroups, 47–49, 72
  of experienced parents, 171
  single-sex, 167–168

Teacher(s)
  as agent of change, 198–202
  aims and approach of, 18–22
  and 'difficult' topics, 188–189,
      193–194, 196–197

Teachers (*cont.*)
  and disabled parents, 179–180
  and ethnic minorities, 180–186
  feedback to, 149, 209–218
  meetings of, 227–228
  motivation of, 17–18
  and presence of fathers, 161–162
  relationship with learner of, 13
  as team, 101–102, 147–151
  and teenage parents, 175
  as visual aid, 133–139
  in working partnership, 221–226
Team-teaching, 147–151
  and relaxation sessions, 101–102
Technology, 195–197, 199
Teenage parents, 173–178
Tension, contrasting relaxation with,
    105–106
Time
  for coverage of topic, 36–37
  for group discussion, 50, 77
  planning of, after birth, 91–92
Topics
  'difficult', 188–197
  new ideas for, 219–220, 227–230
  selection of, 31–35, 45, 50–52
    fathers and, 164–165
  subdivision of, 54–56
  time allocation for, 36–37
Touch
  relaxation, 107, 109
  see also Massage
Training, ongoing, 227–230
Trigger pictures, 89–90

Umbilical cord, model of, 140
Unhelpful behaviour, 78–79

Venue for classes, 14, 40–41, 96–97
Videos, 145, 169
Visual aid(s), 133–146
  fathers and, 169
  teacher's body as, 133–139
Visualization and relaxation, 110–112

Words, choice of, *see* Language
Workshops, 228

Young parents, 173–178